Let Meditation be thy Medicine

THE TIMELESS HEALING WISDOM OF TIBET

Dr. Nida Chenagtsang

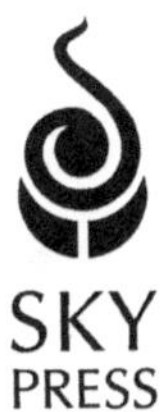

SKY
PRESS

Published by:

Sky Press

Pure Land Farms
3265 Santa Maria Road
Topanga, CA 90290

www.skypressbooks.com

ISBN: 9781950153220

Editor: Katie Malachuk
Design and Typesetting: Pearse Gaffney
First English Edition
Printed on acid-free paper

Special thanks to all whose valuable contributions
made this work possible.

Contents

"Let food be thy medicine
and medicine be thy food."

- Hippocrates of Kos (460 – c. 370 BC)

Author's Preface

Meditation is one of the greatest gifts of ancient human civilization. Today we generally associate the practice of meditation with Asian traditions, but in examining the word itself, we can see that it also has its roots in Western culture. I chose the title *Let Meditation be thy Medicine* to honor the Greek physician Hippocrates, known as the father of Western medicine, and to illustrate the universal and timeless principles of healing.

In Latin, the word *meditatum* means "to ponder"—to focus the mind and ponder about life and to reflect on our inner emotions. How do we ponder? We can find the answer to this question in the ancient Greek tradition in which the word for meditation is *dialogismos*. Each of our internal, multi-layered emotions can get to know each other by dialoguing amongst themselves, and this internal conversation is the most effective way to generate inner peace and harmony within the individual.

The Sanskrit word for meditation, *dhyana*, suggests a movement or flow of the mind without distraction. In Tibetan, the word for meditation is *gom*. *Gom* means "to become familiar with" or "to build a friendship." By becoming familiar with our inner processes, we learn to accept and befriend all aspects of ourselves. The easiest way to build a genuine friendship with ourselves is to breathe. In ancient times, the breath was known as the "spirit" (*spiritus* in Latin). The breath is the bridge between our body and mind, and is the foundation of spirituality.

All of these words show that meditation is a practice that utilizes our active thinking mind—the goal of meditation is not, as many people believe, to become thoughtless and emotionless, but rather to become fully aware of our innermost dimensions. Likewise, we see that meditation is not only a mental process, but involves the physical body and energy as well.

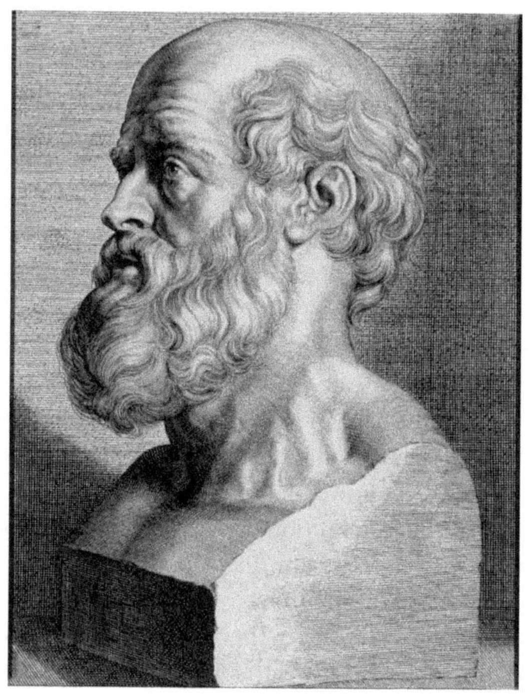

Hippocrates of Kos (460 – c. 370 BC)

We can therefore understand that the final goal of meditation is to find harmony and balance, which is also the goal of Sowa Rigpa (Tibetan Medicine), since the balance of body, energy, and mind is the foundation of good health. How do we achieve this balance and good health? The methods are many and the process begins by getting to know ourselves. By understanding our unique physical, mental, and energetic constitution, we can learn how to best care for and heal ourselves, both spiritually and medically.

This book presents the diverse methods of meditation that have been practiced for centuries by Tibetan yogis and yoginis and teaches you how to find your own unique way within the multitude of methods. As a doctor myself, I see the Buddha as a great physician and psychologist, and his teachings as medicine. This book presents the essential connection between healing and spirituality.

I'd like to thank all those who have made this book possible by bringing my teachings on Sowa Rigpa and the Yuthok Nyingthig into print for a wider audience.

Dr. Nida Chenagtsang
April 2024 in New York

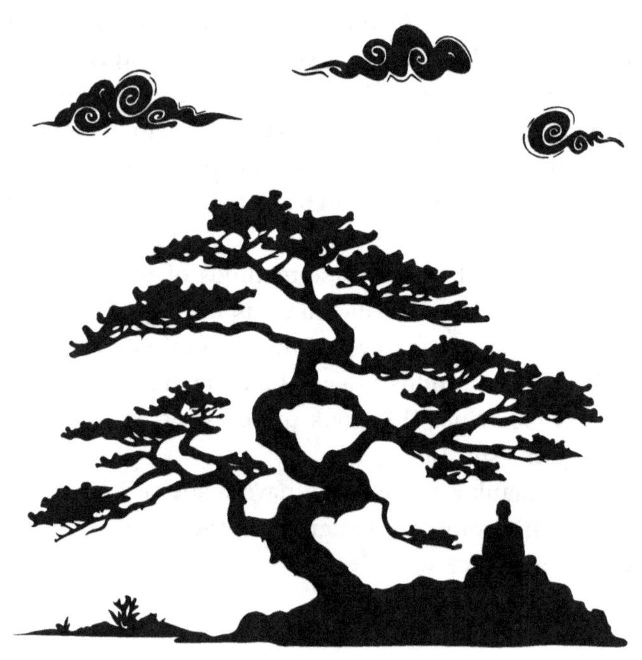

Editor's Preface

It has been a profound honor to work on this book for Dr. Nida Chenagtsang. For a writer and a Tantric Buddhist practitioner, this has felt like a rare form of Guru Yoga.

This book draws most notably from Yuthok's Heart Teachings, an extensive, one-hundred-day retreat and series of teachings offered in 2020, as well as further retreats and conversations with Dr. Nida Chenagtsang from 2022 to 2024.

I am so grateful to Christiana Polites, and Sky Press, for giving me the opportunity to do this work, along with tremendous freedom in how to do it.

I offer my deepest gratitude to Dr. Nida Chenagtsang for trusting me with his words and wisdom. I actually do not have the words to express my appreciation for his generosity. So I will rely upon these most beautiful words that Yuthok gifted to us all:

From whose kindness great bliss itself instantly arises within us,
the guru with jewel-like form, holder of the vajra,
I prostrate at your feet.

Katie Malachuk

"Meditation is a dialogue with ourselves."

- Dr. Nida Chenagtsang

Introduction

Toxins! They seem to be everywhere out there—in our food, our water, our plastics, our relationships. So you try to get rid of them. You eat organic, install filters, bring your own bags, set boundaries with your mother, cut off contact with that ex. But, still, the toxins are there. You can feel them. No matter how much you cleanse and boundary-set, you still feel uncomfortable in your skin and restless in your mind, not to mention affected by illnesses well before old age and obsessed with your traumas and dramas. Why? Because the call is coming from inside the house! The toxins are within. The most powerful toxins—the ones ultimately responsible for polluting our environments and bodies and relationships—are the toxins of the mind.

Over two thousand years ago, the Buddha named these toxins as poisons and diagnosed the big three that infect our minds and lives. Anger. Desire. Ignorance. Many spiritual medicines have been developed to alleviate these poisons—medicines of renunciation, medicines of transformation, different medicines for different kinds of minds and lives and times. About a thousand years ago, a unique Tibetan spiritual teacher and medical doctor, Yuthok Yönten Gönpo, foresaw a time when people would be busy and lazy, too busy and too lazy to utilize many of the medicines of renunciation and transformation. So he developed a path of teachings and practices combining Tibet's two main sciences—Buddhism, the inner science, and Sowa Rigpa, the healing science—to deliver people to overall health as well as spiritual liberation. The main medicine of this path is balance.

It was this emphasis on balance and freedom that first drew me to Yuthok's teachings on medicine and then spirituality. I grew up in a yurt on the grasslands of Amdo, Tibet, living a nomadic lifestyle. I come from a large family—my parents, six brothers, and three sisters. My parents worked very hard, with my father traveling for business and my mother sleeping only four hours a day as she cared for ten children, milked yaks to make butter and cheese, dried yak dung for fire to warm us and cook for us, and sewed all of our clothes. I loved my family, our nomadic existence, and our grasslands, especially the short summers when it indeed became a land of green grass and wild flowers. I felt a deep connection with the flowers and learned the emotional truth, not just the intellectual truth, of impermanence each year when the flowers died after just two precious months of splendor. My family valued education. At seven, I started nomad school. We sat on the floor of a yurt and wrote our lessons with sticks in the dirt. At sixteen, I went to college in the city of Rebkong, which was also beautiful with its tall, naked mountains, but it wasn't my sweet grasslands. One summer, when I was home visiting, I was walking in the flower fields with my father and became overwhelmed with love for these flowers and this place. The beauty of nature is beyond expression. What else are we looking for? It's all here. I felt communication with the flowers and profound peace. I wanted to share this with my father, but it seemed stupid and obvious, though it was bringing me to tears. I knew that in this life I wanted to be connected with nature and plants and flowers, but I didn't know then that Tibetan medicine is connected with nature and plants and flowers.

After college, while I was working as a teacher, a series of serendipitous events led me to take evening classes in Tibetan medicine, known as Sowa Rigpa. Yuthok is the father of Sowa Rigpa, and we were studying the Sowa Rigpa medical tantras, which he is said to have compiled. Tantra has many associations in Western culture, but the word means body protection. So, through Yuthok's teachings and the medical tantras, I was learning how to protect and care for the human body, and I was loving it. I was still quite young, and I was having fun—studying, being with friends, writing poetry, drinking alcohol. One summer, we had a Tibetan medicine herbal camp—hiking in the mountains, living in tents, picking herbs and plants. That moment it all came together for me. This was a path about nature and emotions and balance—and that was exactly what I wanted to do with my life.

Tibetan medicine is deeply connected with Tibetan Buddhism. Though I learned Buddhist teachings growing up, my medical studies inspired a new hunger for spiritual study and practice. So I approached Buddhism in a formal way, as it is traditionally done—I sought out teachers.

I was fortunate to encounter humble, powerful, learned teachers from the main schools of Tibetan Buddhism; some were more practice focused and some were more study focused. While I was working and going to medical school, I traveled each weekend to see my teachers. I brought them food. I requested teachings. I was turned down sometimes. I received teachings. I stayed in monasteries. I meditated in caves. I considered becoming a monastic. Though most of my teachers were monastics, they helped me see that my path was that of the ngakpa—the non-monastic, non-celibate yogi. And, indeed, I would go on to be a yogi householder with a family. In the Tibetan Buddhist tradition, the monastics and yogis are all tantric practitioners but with different sets of vows depending on their focus in this lifetime. As we will discuss, the tantric path helps people discover and use their strengths as sources of health and growth. In this way, spiritual paths are very personal; they are based on karmic connections and individual inclinations. With my inner pull toward nature and balance, it made sense for me to be a yogi where not only the inner cultivation but also the outer expression is that of the natural human state. As will also be discussed, the tantric spiritual approach emphasizes that we are naturally balanced and, as such, blissful. However, we have become imbalanced through various patterns and influences within and around us; thus, we are suffering. The yogis are often recognized by their long hair and white clothing, all of which represent the primordially pure and balanced and blissful state of being we are uncovering through practice—no matter what we wear or how we appear.

While I was studying the Sowa Rigpa medical tantras, I heard about Yuthok's other book—the Yuthok Nyingthig, or Yuthok's heart-essence teachings, which is mainly a spiritual text. I wanted to read it, but I felt I didn't have enough time. Again, in addition to being a medical student, I was so spiritually excited that I was jumping from text to text, doing different practices, studying with many teachers. But my medical teachers kept telling us that the Yuthok Nyingthig would be practical when we were practicing medicine. We wouldn't have time to do long spiritual practices and retreats, and the Yuthok Nyingthig is uniquely essentialized, easy to practice, and effective. I listened to this, but I didn't really hear it. However, when I finally had the opportunity and desire to do a seven-day retreat of the Yuthok Nyingthig practices, something changed for me in a meditative way. I felt the blessing of Yuthok as a master who connected everything. It helped me understand all the other teachings I was receiving. It helped me understand everything.

As humans, it is normal for us to separate into groups or schools or sects and then think our way is different from others and also perfect. Yuthok helped me see all buddhas as one buddha, all gurus as one guru. He tells us not to chase after teachings and practices. We need to know the essence of the teachings. Theoretically, it made sense. Then, when I did his practices, something clicked. I went from being a young scholar, thinking this way, my way, was the best way to instead being totally relaxed. I could see all teachings as one, just coming from different angles and aspects. It was very powerful. It made me more flexible. Before I had critical ideas about this or that because I was ignorant. We think we are smart and special when we look for difference and compare ideas to say what is better than others. But it is really smart and special to see how they are all connected, all in one. Then we are more balanced and closer to our natural state of bliss.

I was also drawn to Yuthok because who he was as a person and what he shared as a teacher felt especially suited for this time. Yuthok was a family man who balanced his spiritual practice and teachings with a robust medical practice. Of course, he showed all the signs that such spiritual masters do, such as visions of buddhas as well as miraculous events surrounding him, especially during teachings. Still, he maintained his focus on medicine, becoming an unparalleled physician, even the royal physician, and donating medicines as well as clothing and food to those in need. Also, because he was involved with his children as a father, with his wife as a husband, with his students as a teacher, with his patients as a doctor, he understood human psychology from many access points. For example, once a king had eye problems and sought Yuthok's guidance. Yuthok examined the king's eyes and said, "The problem is not with your eyes; it is that your tail is growing." The king replied, "I don't want a tail!" So Yuthok told him to massage his tail every day. After a few days, the king's eye problem cleared. He told Yuthok he had been massaging his tail every day, but then he had to wash his hands. Yuthok had known that the real issue was the king's hands were dirty when he was touching his eyes, but the king would have felt embarrassed had Yuthok initially told him to wash his hands. This is one of countless stories where Yuthok displayed his creativity, humanity, and pragmatism. And he used these qualities to develop a spiritual path that focuses on efficient practices and fast blessings. He saw that in his time people did not have much time for spirituality, and life was only going to be faster in the future. So he did not give many philosophical teachings. He gave short, crucial lessons and practices, and I have found that they give us exactly what we need right now.

Mostly, in the Buddhist tradition, spiritual masters are monastics. They are doing the wonderful work of preserving the tradition perfectly, passing it carefully from generation to generation like an antique. This is extremely important and necessary work. However, as monastics, they often manage their emotions a bit differently than laypeople. They don't suffer as much with family relationships. They don't know about heartbreak, which is one of our main issues as laypeople. Because Yuthok was also a layperson and a doctor, he wasn't focused on preserving the tradition like an antique; he was focused on serving the patient in front of him. He was willing to improvise with the antidote based on the cause of the suffering. Classical training is always important, but sometimes jazz hits the spot. Recently, I was talking with a Tibetan geshe, where I live in Italy, who said that Italians are crazy. He recounted how a man came to him and said of his partner, "I hate this woman. We have so many problems, and now I am very sad." The woman came to the geshe and said, "I hate this man; he is a very bad man." For the geshe, it is easy. The man thinks the woman is bad, and the woman thinks the man is bad—then separate. But we know the problem—they're in love. The geshe doesn't understand that kind of entanglement. For him, this is stupid; just cut it and that's it. Maybe this geshe has never fallen in love; he has never experienced this heartache. And, in one way, the geshe is absolutely right, and some people may be able to break up like that. But, in other ways, there's a possible lack of understanding, and there may be skillful means to work with this couple to preserve the union and their happiness. Yuthok understood these things and adapted his spiritual teachings and medical practice for ordinary humans in their time and place.

So here we find ourselves with the age-old human problem of mental toxins and myriad teachings to address them. However, we have limited time and energy in our busy and lazy lives. Therefore, Yuthok presented a simple but completely accurate way of understanding and then addressing our disease. What Yuthok knew, as a teacher and a doctor, is that these mental toxins are the result of imbalances in your body, energy, and mind. In fact, these so-called toxins are nothing more than your organic elemental makeup that is currently messed up. As has long been taught in the Buddhist tradition, everything in our world, including your body, energy, and mind, is made up of the five elements—space, wind, fire, earth, and water—in different proportions. Because everything is born from space, and we are busy and lazy, Yuthok says we can focus on wind, fire, and earth/water. Most of us have one predominate element, maybe two. Thanks to predominance and imbalance, the elements take on toxic qualities in your mind that cause suffering for you and everyone around you and the entire world. This is not the mind manifesting illness or pain or misfortune in a magical woo-woo way. This is basic cause and effect. So let's take a walk through the cause-and-effect process of suffering for fire, wind, and earth/water imbalance as it all looks and sounds today—inviting the examples and voices of countless patients and students, compiled with love in a fiercely compassionate case-study way.

Let's say you have an imbalance of fire. You're a hothead. You're angry. You're pissed. You feel like it's you versus everyone. You feel victim-y, even narcissistic-y, seduced by stories of your martyrdom. You're right and they're wrong; you hurt and they are to blame. Your boiling mind boils life down to aggrieved me versus annoying other. You need to let off some steam, maybe pick a fight or punch a wall, take a drink or smoke a bowl, run a marathon or lay some lovers.

Maybe you did pick fights in your youth or relished really aggressive athletic competition. Maybe that left you with nagging injuries in your joints or sticky thought loops of regret or revenge or resentment. Maybe you're clenching your jaw and grinding your teeth, getting headaches, and having diarrhea. Maybe you're drawn to angry and violent movies or news or conversations. Maybe you obsess over protecting yourself or protecting others or harming yourself or harming others, and making plans to do so, even carrying them out. Maybe it makes sense to have some weapons because you never know when shit is gonna go down, and you can be the hero or the villain, either would be justified. Maybe you seek out political groups that use divisive speech or even violence, and you send your votes and dollars in directions that keep large-scale fighting going for us all.

Maybe you found that alcohol would quench the fire or weed would snuff it out. Maybe the substances that kept you out of worse trouble then became your keeper. Maybe it's difficult to stick with a stable job or relationship; you're struggling with money and loneliness. Or maybe you're pulling it all off somehow. You can't have a problem if you still have a job or family, right? It's just a little mommy juice or daddy grass, and you have freaking earned it because life is so hard. After all, your choices were hardly choices with all that pressure and expectation, right? Maybe your sleep is restless and your digestion is out of whack, and you're feeling inflamed and nauseous. Maybe you have some chest pain, but that couldn't be because you're too young. Maybe in your self-medicated haze you give fewer fucks about everything, and isn't that the goal these days? Why give a damn about anyone else if they don't give a damn about you? Why pay attention to how you participate in your community or vote with your dollars? It's not your problem because you have enough going on. Just do whatever it takes to take the edge off the very hard slog of being you.

Maybe you quit the fights after high school and dropped the substances after a messy few years and then returned to sports, the call of your youth. You started running. You can outrun the anger. You can burn out the heat. You just need to keep going. You can do marathons, even ultramarathons. Maybe your knees are giving way, so you get a sweet bike and hit the pool and now you can do triathlons. As long as you can train, you have a reason to get up each day and crush it. Maybe it's not only your knees but also your perineum now that the bike's involved. Maybe something's up with your orgasm, too, like you're coming too quickly or lightly, like a flame flickering, but how can that be when you're in killer shape and look super hot? Maybe your partner is getting tired of picking up the slack because you're training all the time, and when you're not training you're on your phone because you're crushing it at work, too. Maybe you ditched the partner because they were slowing you down in so many ways, and now you're crushing the dating apps. Text this one, hit up that one, hook up with that one. Good thing you've got a good memory. But maybe no matter how many partners, positions, or toys you try, your orgasm is still flickery and you're never satisfied. Maybe you're buying fancier this and that because you look so good and deserve so much and you're freaked out about your orgasm and who cares about consumerism. Maybe you're racking up flights here, there, and everywhere to train and race and work and chill and who cares about carbon footprint. Maybe you're making everything into a competition, and your kid is tired of it and everyone around you as well because you're exhausting.

Maybe you've tried meditation. But it's hard to sit still, and your mind won't settle down. Besides you have a lot going on. Maybe you need to outsource meditation. You listen to that meditation app for a few minutes before bed or listen to that podcast about meditating while you're driving. That counts, right? Plus, it gives you stuff to think about on your runs and talk about on your dates. Maybe you're thinking about microdosing, like everyone in your social media feed, so you can stay on top of your game.

Or, let's say you have an imbalance of wind. Your head is in the clouds. You are floating above it all, only deigning to touch down for desire. Sometimes you want to do this and sometimes you want to do that. Sometimes you want to be here and sometimes you want to be there. Sometimes you want to kiss this one and sometimes you want to kiss that one. Mostly you want to be free—and safe. Because it's all a lot. And you're blowing in the breeze. You need to find some ground, have a moment, take a breath. Or maybe not, because being is boring, and you are ready to fly into your fantasies where all your wishes are fulfilled.

Maybe you have always known how to fly—with your mind. You know how to fly away from the disappointments of this place. You can fly into your imagination, where your dreams and desires are realized—a world of beauty and love and perfection and everything you've ever wanted. There, you get the girl, the guy, the prize, the praise. Maybe you spend most of your days daydreaming—staring out the window, wanting. You're creative; that's what you've realized. So creative, so talented. Of course, you're an artist. And misunderstood. Possibly a bit tortured. Unrecognized for your brilliance. Because your art and creativity, it's all so special. You're before your time, beyond your time, beyond all time—and space. Life's categories and expectations want to pin you down. But you can't be pinned down. You can't even sleep. And when you finally do sleep, you have nightmares. How dare they interfere with your daydreams? Maybe you're also aging kind of fast, which doesn't align with your fantasized future of beauty and love and perfection forevermore. How could you be aging when your real life hasn't even begun? You wish you had someone to talk to, all the time, but you don't want anyone to know that because you're supposed to be above it all, beyond it all. And here you are online shopping at 3 a.m. For what? You forgot.

Maybe you are actually anxious and fearful and farting all the time. Underneath all that creativity and fantasy and imagination, underneath all those songs and poems and scripts and witticisms is a mind too scared to be in this moment because there is too much to feel. And you have no idea how to be still with it all. Even worse, there is so much that could go wrong, or at least wrong in that it doesn't align with your attachments and plans and concepts about what's right. Maybe you are aging fast because you are constantly thinking, often worrying, about yourself and everyone else. Maybe you develop compulsions to avoid your thinking or assuage your worrying. Drinking and smoking? Sure. Drugs and shopping? Of course. But maybe your favorites are seducing and scrolling—preferably at the same time. Let's send songs and sun signs and soar off into space. No need to get serious and make a mess. Keep it open and light and never never land. Who cares how it affects others? Who even cares how it affects you? Maybe it's all an illusion anyway. And maybe, just maybe, your precious artistry is another addiction. Maybe you are actually spreading compulsive thinking through your supposed creativity. Maybe with your anxiety masquerading as artistry you are infecting others' minds with your inability to be. Maybe that's too terrifying to think about because then what? Who are you without your interesting thoughts? What is life without your precious daydreams?

Maybe instead of worrying about the big questions you just worry about leaving the house. Seeing as you already feel a little unsafe in your skin, your safest bet is to stay in the daydream world where it all works out and nothing can hurt you. Because maybe you already feel hurt, not only emotionally and existentially but also physically, like all over. Maybe there's pain in your lower back, pain in your pelvis, pain in your feet, pain here and pain there. The pain migrates like your mind, blowing this way and that. Being alive kind of hurts. Maybe all of life hurts. You have tried to leave the house. You have tried so hard to do the stuff of this world. You have tried to be good and pure and perfect. You have tried to please this person and that person. You have tried to help. You are always trying to help. No one understands how much you are trying to help. They even get angry with you for trying to help. You have done all you can, and still you don't get what you want—not the girl, not the guy, not the prize, not the praise. All you get is constipation. Maybe the real problem is you can never get what you want. You can see it in your mind, in your daydreams, in your heart of hearts. You're a walking vision board. But it never works out like you imagine—even the girl, the guy, the prize, the praise. No wonder you're sensitive and moody and unstable. How can you be expected to keep being nice and cheerful and funny and creative after all you've done to do it all right only to end up feeling all wrong.

Maybe you've tried meditation. But it turns into a trip to fantasy island, or an hour of to-do listing, or a songwriting session. Are you really supposed to let all of those brilliant, creative ideas float on by? No, you're picking up your pen and putting all that awesome down on paper. Today, you'll perfect your manifesting and your manuscript. You can start your meditation practice tomorrow.

Or, let's say you have an imbalance of earth/water. You bury your head in the sand. And your lack of awareness is the perfect breeding ground for ignorance in all its forms. Life involves so much this and that, and who cares. You are checked out, tuned out, zoned out, spaced out. What you don't know can't hurt you, so you stay safely out of the fray. You sit back and take it easy. Let everyone else do the runaround and blah blah blah—you are stuck in the mud.

Maybe it would feel good to actually be in mud, like a mud bath. Maybe you can't get enough of sensation all over your skin, the thicker and heavier and wetter the better. You could stay in that mud all day, like a super spa day, feeling that warm weight envelop you and cocoon you and pull you down into sleep. You could sleep forever. Waking up is so hard. Maybe the only thing harder than waking up is getting out of bed. Maybe you love to hang out in the slip of your sheets, under the heft of your blankets, the sensation of snuggling in, all safe and cozy and nothing to do. Maybe you masturbate there for even more sensation, then fall back asleep. Maybe the only thing that pulls you from bed is the thought of breakfast. Maybe food is your true love. Oh, the sensation of eating food—the smells, the textures, the tastes, the look of it just before you dig in, the feeling of chewing and chewing and chewing, the sweetness of fullness, the satiety of stuffed. Maybe the only thing better than sleeping is feasting. Or fucking. Feasting with genitals—brilliant. A long session of fucking, followed by massive feasting, then endless sleeping. Chef's kiss! But you're a connoisseur, of course, of all these things. You are a sensual artist. You are not looking for banal binges. You want to soak up every sense pleasure, slowly and fully. You are a foodie, a gourmand. You are a lover extraordinaire. You are bedding down in the best of accoutrements. You'll get your work done; you're reliable. But why bring up work at a moment like this? Life is so delicious. Who can blame you for wanting to take everything in?

Maybe in taking everything in, you are shutting everything out. Maybe your physical pleasure palace is actually a comfort zone of control where you hide from the world. Maybe you sleep away your entire morning in those satin sheets because you don't want to deal. Maybe your steadfast reliability becomes stubborn monotony, and your colleagues and friends and family feel it. Maybe you are a stone sinking to the bottom as lethargy drags you under, and you are in denial about your descent into depression. Maybe those foodie foods start losing their flavor, and you over-salt and over-sweeten to taste anything at all. Gourmand be gone, as your lack of taste and lack of energy compels you to eat whatever you can get your hands on. Maybe your charmingly curvy and beautifully buoyant body morphs into something that doesn't feel or look like you, but maybe you don't even notice. You're too consumed with consuming, desperately seeking sensation in a futile attempt to pierce through your increasingly numbed out body and mind. Maybe you make your way to weed—a perfect fit as the numbed finds the numbing. At least being high makes you hungry, giving you an excuse to rip it open and bring on the binge. Of course, the only thing better than shoving food into your face is shoving food into your face while staring into a screen. Social media and gaming give you the illusion that you are participating in something called life. In reality, you are numbing deeper and deeper. Maybe you turn to more violent games or shows to shock yourself into feeling. Maybe you turn to violence toward yourself or others to shock yourself into feeling alive. Maybe it hasn't occurred to you what any of this means for those around you. You could try getting laid though it's unlikely you can get aroused. And, if you do find the energy to get some sex, maybe your partners feel like you're consuming them instead of connecting with them. You'd like to poop for relief, and possibly some godforsaken pleasure, but even that is escaping you these days. Maybe you don't even notice that your kid is looking out the window at you, wondering why you are always in the backyard, as you smoke another spliff. Maybe you don't see that your partner is hitting their rock bottom because whenever they look to you, you are looking at your phone. Maybe you've stopped considering the consequences as you toss back edibles and get behind the wheel of a car, your toddler buckled up in back and countless others sharing the highway with you.

Maybe you don't realize that by sinking into yourself you are moving in direct opposition to realization. Because when you focus on your experience—your body, your senses, your mind, your story, your pain—you forget the reality of team effort. Maybe you think that if you stay out of the way, you aren't part of the story. Maybe you think that if you don't look too closely, then you aren't responsible for it. Maybe you have forgotten that everything affects everything and we are all responsible for all of it. Maybe you haven't encountered teachings on the wisdom of interdependence, but regardless you understand the suffering of being sucked into yourself. You see how ignorance gives rise to anger and desire as you cling to self-centeredness at all costs. But maybe you are not yet ready to release self-absorption in the same way your body can't release the fluids pooling in your feet. You are stuck in physical and mental edema, holding on for your life, not knowing that living begins when you release me for we.

Maybe you have tried meditation. But you just go to sleep. It all seems like so much freaking work. And for what? Nothing changes. Besides, between your high thoughts and the occasional trip, aren't you pretty much enlightened already?

If any of that sounded at all familiar to you, welcome to being a human being. We are all in the toxic stew together. You need never be ashamed or afraid of your human mind. These mental spins and assorted sufferings are simply the result of being imbalanced, and balance can always be restored. In fact, the pull toward balance is instinctive to your humanness and also the path to your liberation and potential to be of great benefit to us all. You organically know how to care for yourself and others and our world.

Indeed, the origin story of the Sowa Rigpa medical tantras provides us with an example of our deep knowing of health and freedom. While it was Yuthok who is said to have compiled the four medical tantras of Sowa Rigpa, they were initially birthed into being through Medicine Buddha. As you will come to know more and more through this book, a buddha is just like you, but balanced. Medicine Buddha exists in a state of complete harmony and liberation, free from the three poisons of ignorance, desire, and anger. As the story goes, Medicine Buddha sat in single-pointed meditation, and his single point of focus was to heal all beings from all suffering. So he asked himself how to do this. Specifically, his throat chakra asked his heart chakra. An internal dialogue began, and, ultimately, the throat chakra elicited responses from the head, heart, navel, and root chakras to create the four medical tantras that prevent illness, cure illness, extend life, and cultivate happiness.

We can relate to this story because nearly all the time we have a hungry aspect of mind that is asking questions, wanting things, wondering what to do, and making plans. And sometimes, when we are relaxed and balanced, we have a wise aspect of mind that provides clear, calm, loving, and compassionate guidance to us. Actually, the Greek word for meditation is dialogismos—meditation is a dialogue with ourselves. However, we are usually consumed by ignorance, desire, and anger and their runoffs of pride and jealousy such that our questions, thoughts, and contemplations are muddled and self-serving. Nor are we focused, relaxed, or balanced enough for our inherent wisdom to dialogue with us and guide us into compassionate activity of body, speech, and mind. Medicine Buddha was able to birth the extraordinarily compassionate creation of the medical tantras because of his single-pointed focus on benefiting beings, which was made possible by his perfect wisdom, also known as the absence of ignorance, desire, and anger. This wisdom and compassion is inherently available to all of us when we find elemental balance and release our mental toxins. It is entirely within your capabilities to uncover health and happiness across all aspects of your life. Indeed, you can promote not only health and happiness but also ease and freedom for yourself and others.

Thanks to the blessings of Medicine Buddha and Yuthok, this book presents a path to balance, well-being, and freedom. There are multitudes of medicines available to us through Yuthok's two treasures—the medical tantras and his heart-essence spiritual teachings. As a practitioner and teacher of Sowa Rigpa, I have other books that focus more on the medical teachings of Yuthok, including diet and lifestyle modifications, herbal medications, and bodywork. However, I am also a lineage holder of Yuthok's spiritual teachings, so I teach his heart-essence practices and prescribe spiritual remedies as well. In talking with countless students and patients, I have seen time and time again the common and unfortunate misunderstanding that spiritual practice is one size fits all. Nothing could be further from the truth. There are so many spiritual options for working with the body, speech-energy, and mind. In fact, we are often helped by different spiritual practices at different times depending on our elemental makeup during different periods of our lives. So, in this book, I will briefly touch on diet and lifestyle modifications, but I will focus on spiritual practices and how to apply them depending on your elemental makeup.

In Chapter One, we will explore the common Buddhist metaphor of suffering as the disease, the Buddha as the doctor, and the path as the medicine. This will give us the opportunity to look more closely at the pain and confusion of elemental imbalance as well as how teachers and a spiritual path can help to heal us. Also, we will look at where Yuthok and his teachings fit within the Buddhist tradition so we feel grounded as we start to step onto this path. In Chapter Two, we will look at Yuthok's two treasures. We will take a walk through the Yuthok Nyingthig, his heart-essence spiritual teachings, and we will briefly discuss Sowa Rigpa so that you can engage in an elemental typology self-assessment to determine whether you are a wind, fire, or earth/water type. In Chapters Three, Four, and Five, we will look at spiritual practices that are well suited for wind, fire, and earth/water types respectively and also discuss some diet and lifestyle modifications. Ideally, you will come to better know yourself and how to balance yourself—as balance across body, energy, and mind is the very definition of health and freedom. These days there is increasing research showing that meditation can improve mental and physical well-being; this book will help you understand how this is possible.

Before we dive into this healing journey, allow me to offer a powerful motivational supplement. Recall from the story of Medicine Buddha that his single-pointed focus on benefiting beings allowed him to reveal remedies for all of our ills. As you approach the teachings in this book, perhaps the most powerful medicine available to you is to consider the two aims of self and other—meaning, once you address your imbalance, how can you ultimately apply this knowledge to be of benefit to others? This motivation is powerful medicine because the most poisonous and toxic thing you do is think about yourself all the time.

"These practices do not add anything;
they reveal what is already there."

- Dr. Nida Chenagtsang

Chapter One – The View

Often when you hear serious spiritual practitioners talk about their teachers, they do so with great reverence, even devotion. This happens naturally, out of gratitude, because our teachers help us to establish right view—and this is the true start of a spiritual path. Stepping onto a spiritual path is not about changing your outfit or name or hairstyle or home or any external this and that. Stepping onto a spiritual path is about changing your view.

Right view means the honest, organic truths of being human. It is the foundation that gives rise to compassionate creativity and altruistic responsiveness as displayed in right thought, right speech, and right action. Wrong view builds up our mental toxins of ignorance, desire, and anger as well as pride and jealousy. With wrong view, everything goes wrong—thoughts, speech, actions, all promoting negativity, conflict, strife, and stress. Right view brings long-term happiness and good health and balance, within us and among us. And it is already present in your mind. Buried under all of your wrong and confused views is right view, just waiting to be realized.

The thing is, most human beings are like bonsai trees, living in little pots made of conditioned views. This is good, at first. This is safe. Our parents and caregivers put us in a safe, little pot. Our roots get covered with different layers of dirt that have been passed down over generations—layers of culture, layers of custom, layers of tradition, layers of education, layers of religion, layers of concepts about what humans can and can't do. We grow in our pots and sit next to each other at kindergarten in our little pots. Over the years, we are shaped and pruned and molded like beautiful little bonsai trees. We are so cute. Little bonsais, told what to wear, what to do, how to be a girl, how to be a boy. Then we go in our little pots to high school and college and work. Maybe when we left our childhood home we were removed from a pot and put in a park, but we still didn't truly open. Our roots are still in a little ball—our neurons traveling down paths trained in pots. We are still showered and clean, so to speak, even as we try on different outfits, even spiritual outfits. As bonsais, we are mostly focused on our appearance. We are all made up—following dress codes of whatever culture we want to follow. We could be tidy-looking bonsais or sloppy-looking bonsais or spiritual-looking bonsais. Or, uh oh, maybe we are ikebana, without even roots; maybe we are dressed up in artificial perfection. Bonsai and ikebana are beautiful as art. The leaves and flowers are gorgeous. But no one is thinking about the roots—they are wrapped and bound and even cut. So we become drawn to artificial and superficial things because we are artificial and superficial ourselves. No matter our age or appearance, we are bonsai and ikebana, conforming to cultural or even countercultural norms.

Maybe it is good, at first, to be bonsai. As kids, we needed the safety of the pot; we needed structure and containment to get rooted. But then our root balls felt cramped by our pots. Our roots became entangled, bound, and rigid. We became entangled, bound, and rigid. We can feel it, and it feels wrong. We want to stretch our roots, our minds, beyond what we see culturally and counterculturally and even spiritually. To do this, we need to leave our bonsai pots. We need to become free. So we enter the forest. Because humans, like trees, do not belong in pots. We want to have roots and minds that can stretch—free and clear to flow with nutrients and information. But, having been in a pot, we now need teachers to help us navigate the forest.

We may think we don't need teachers. We may think we can go it alone in the forest. This makes sense because we're adults. We're cooking, working, paying bills, perhaps raising a family of our own. But to get to this place of caregiving for self and others, we needed parents and teachers and mentors who taught us everything from how to wipe our butts to how to make breakfast to how to bring in income. These people taught us the ways of the world. Some of us had parents and caregivers who did this very well, and some of us may not have had these people. There is no doubt that parents and caregivers love their children, but they do not always have the tools they need to teach their children well. Maybe they don't know how to express their love. Maybe they don't know how to educate their children. Maybe they are lacking an open mind about options for their children's futures. Maybe they want to protect their children because they themselves were not protected. Maybe they want to treat their children like a little prince or princess, even though the world won't treat them this way. Maybe they want to create a perfect and cozy place for their children at home, even though the world is not perfect or cozy. Maybe they think what is right for them is what is right for their children. So maybe we learned what we needed from our parents and caregivers and maybe we did not. Either way, we probably looked beyond our parents and caregivers and found additional teachers and mentors who helped us learn more about how to live in the world. We have gone to school; we have learned on the job. Humans need help to develop our worldly lives.

It is the same on the spiritual path. At some point, most humans seek out a spiritual path even if that means rejecting a spiritual path. Path and no path are both paths. Maybe some of us received spiritual instruction as children, or maybe not. Either way, we need to do our own exploration and develop our own spiritual path whether it aligns with our families and communities or not. Spiritual paths are very personal. When we develop our personal spiritual path, as adults, we again need teachers. Even though we are older in body and mind, we still need someone to start from the beginning with us to teach us how to wipe our spiritual butts. We don't need fancy or fussy or academic teachers in the forest of spirituality. We already have too much superficiality in our lives. We are mentally unwell and imbalanced and overly emotional and tired of these pots and outfits and expectations. We are looking to be relaxed and organic, like the forest. We need teachers who are relaxed and organic and human style. We need these teachers to tell us the truth of the forest. We need these teachers to introduce us to right view. And right view is not always gentle. It's about transmitting true wisdom and intelligence, and, depending on how we have learned to live in the world, this can feel difficult or disruptive or wild or even offensive. Because uncovering right view is about discovering true freedom. When you begin to see this view and taste this freedom, you realize you are receiving the medicine to release your mental toxins. Though your parents gave you life, and you should be tremendously thankful for this gift, your spiritual teachers are often the doctors who save your life.

In this chapter, you will be introduced to contemplations that can establish right view. These medicines of thinking meditation have been passed down from the original doctor in this tradition, the Buddha. For thousands of years, these medicines have helped people start their spiritual journeys on good footing. These medicines are not more information to put into your mind. Rather, these medicines are about cultivating discernment and recovering your natural intelligence, creativity, and responsiveness. They can help you see your life and mind clearly, allowing you to navigate the forest of freedom with confidence and joy. There is nothing to adopt here, only opportunities to explore. The doctors simply offer the medicine. It is entirely your choice if, when, and how to take it.

THE FOUR THOUGHTS THAT TURN THE MIND

The first medicine on this path is Ngöndro, which means preliminary practice. There are three Ngöndros—common, uncommon, and routine. Because they are styled to specific cycles of teachings, we will talk about the uncommon Ngöndro and routine Ngöndro in the next chapter when we talk more about the Yuthok Nyingthig practice path. However, the common Ngöndro is where we all start because it is meant for any kind of spiritual practitioner and leads one to reflect upon the meaning of life and see its true value. This foundation is important for new and experienced practitioners.

Most of us want to avoid preliminary practices because no one wants to say they are a beginner. But, again, think about your childhood. Maybe it was completely healthy—mentally, emotionally, and physically. If that was the case, then, as you have become an adult, you feel balanced. You set and reach goals. Your goals feel aligned with your true callings. You love your work, have a solid and steady income, and donate most of your money except to provide for basic necessities. You have had nothing but stable and loving friendships and romantic relationships. You care for your mind and body. Your eating is stress free and so is your pooping. You maintain a healthy and consistent body weight. You have a positive body image. Your sexuality and sex life flow without hang-ups. Your orgasms come easily and plentifully. You are free of addictions to substances, food, stuff, or technology. You are free of toxic thoughts. You have no nightmares. You can sit in meditation endlessly with ease. You are comfortable in any crowd and also with silence and solitude. So on and so forth. Chances are this is not the case. Chances are your childhood was not completely healthy. Everyone's childhood includes traumas and dramas. Everyone's childhood could be a book. So probably your childhood included storms. These storms created turbulence in your teenage years. And aspects of your adult life are still turbulent. From the storms of childhood, clouds go on and on and on through you, through your children, through their children.

Giving yourself a good spiritual foundation through Ngöndro is like giving yourself a good spiritual childhood. Ngöndro establishes a good relationship with your spiritual practice. You like the practice. You want to do the practice. Ngöndro even clears obstacles to practice so the rest of your spiritual path is easy and healthy. If you think you don't need Ngöndro and skip it, you will create an unstable foundation, encounter obstacles and resistance, and your spiritual path will not flow. If you have spiritual pride and think you are above Ngöndro, this is a form of confusion that will result in issues in your spiritual development. Starting with the foundation of Ngöndro creates a healthy spiritual childhood for the rest of your practice path and life.

The common Ngöndro involves contemplating four thoughts. These are usually translated as the Four Thoughts that Turn the Mind. I like to call them the Four U-Turn Thoughts because they turn the mind from wrong view to right view.

Precious Human Life

Do you feel your life is precious? Are you sure? How much do you value your life on a scale of one to ten? Be honest. Maybe when everything is going your way, it feels like eight or nine. Maybe when you are experiencing heartbreak or financial stress or illness or addiction or aimlessness or loneliness, it feels like one or even zero. Maybe these days we think a lot about the value of our things or jobs or relationships or appearances or reputations, but not the value of our lives. Maybe we equate our lives with our things or jobs or relationships or appearances or reputations. If we don't see the value of our lives, our basic human existence, we can get very depressed. We may think negatively about ourselves and society and everything. When you think life is bad and negative, you get stuck. You think you are worthless, hopeless, helpless. When you see no value in something, you want to drop it. When you feel there is no value in your life, you may think suicidal thoughts. Those are toxic thoughts—loaded with mental poisons, especially ignorance. We all go there at some point. And, at that point, if you can turn your mind from wanting to end your life to appreciating your life, that is a U-turn from wrong view to right view. Then you really take spirituality seriously because your spiritual path encourages you to find meaning for your life—beyond things or jobs or relationships or appearance or reputation. Your spiritual path helps you see your life in a different way. It gives your life spiritual purpose—such as cultivating overall wellness and contentment for yourself, your family, others, and our world.

Traditionally, on the Buddhist path, it is taught that human lives are a precious opportunity to wake up, as the Buddha did, to complete wholeness, ease, and liberation, to be entirely free of mental toxins and the pain they create for ourselves and others, to instead bring loving kindness and compassion and joy and equanimity to ourselves and others. In fact, it is taught that human life contains just the right amount of suffering and agency to see that a U-turn needs to be made and to make it. Examine this for yourself. If you have the inclination and time to read this book and contemplate these teachings, it is evidence that you have experienced enough suffering to seek greater well-being and meaning in your life and also that you have enough motivation and space to do so. This is a precious situation.

Further, you can consider how amazing it is that you are even here to do this in the first place. You can think about all of the pieces of the puzzle that had to come together for you to be here, right now, reading this book—all of the steps in your ancestral path that aligned for you to exist; all of the experiences requiring myriad causes and conditions involving countless people and materials and synchronicities for you to have grown up, been sheltered, fed, educated, and had the pleasures and sorrows to arrive in this moment; all of the other humans who have studied and practiced and taught these teachings for this information to appear in this book; and so on and so forth. When you pause and contemplate the interdependence involved in this moment, or any moment, it is nothing short of a miracle that you are here right now with the time and space and inclination and motivation to do something that could be of benefit to yourself and everyone around you. It is a precious and valuable opportunity—this life of yours. So, if you would like, please consider how you could honor this gift. You could think about this for a few minutes each day as medicine for your mind.

Impermanence

How often do you think about impermanence? How often do you really think about impermanence? The theory of impermanence is easy to understand. Oh, yes, everything is changing. But sometimes the most accessible theories are the most difficult to practice. We know impermanence theoretically. We see it and experience it. But we don't completely accept it, especially when it comes to our lives. That's the problem. It is ignorant to ignore our impending death; this denial is a confused and toxic mental state. It is wrong view. We know we were born. We know we are alive. We know we will die. Death is part of life. We cannot ignore death. Death is coming. Death is like tomorrow. We don't ignore tomorrow. We save some food for tomorrow. We save some work for tomorrow. We make plans to meet friends tomorrow. We know tomorrow will come. This is also true of death. We don't know at what age—this year, next year, in thirty years? But we will all die. If you think more about impermanence, this inspires a U-turn from confusion and laziness to clarity and purpose. We can no longer say, "I'll do retreat next year. I'll do practice another time. I'll meditate tomorrow. I'm young. I'm healthy." Young can die before old. Healthy can die before sick. There is no guarantee. We know our birth date, but we do not know our death date. We never know which comes first—tomorrow or death. We know tomorrow is coming, and we will enter into tomorrow. In the same way, we know death is coming, and we will enter into death. With wrong view, when death comes, you get scared and panic, and you realize you have wasted your life on meaningless and trivial pursuits, trying to acquire things and relationships that you cannot take with you into death. With right view, you consistently cultivate a peaceful and joyful mental state, which you will take into death and beyond. If you really know each day could be your last, you want to do essential and meaningful things that are actually beneficial for yourself and others. The preliminary practice helps us to live in reality with right view. We have to be in the real world, real life, and this means truly knowing that everyone you love and you will die.

If we think more about our death and the deaths of others, we better understand that death is a natural part of human life and relationships. Then thinking about impermanence also leads to a U-turn from toxic heartache or anger or desire to healthy gratitude. When we lose family and friends and lovers to death or distance or breakups, we feel pain because we do not accept the situation. If you absolutely understand impermanence, it is impossible to have a broken heart. Your heart is breaking because you loved that person and now you have lost them. You might feel hopeless and stuck, wanting things to be as they were. But life can no longer be that way. It is only because of impermanence that you knew and loved that person. Also, what did that loved one want for you when they were alive or when you were together? They wanted you to be happy. I lost my mother a few years ago. I know that she wants me to be happy and to pursue purpose and joy in my life. There is no reason for me to stay stuck in sadness; that is not what we want for our loved ones or what they want for us. Relationships are impermanent. Love stories are impermanent. We can value family and friendship and love, and also understand and accept that all of these connections are impermanent. This is right view. Otherwise, love of all kinds causes so much suffering because of wrong view—we don't understand and accept that love is always impermanent. Each time your heart breaks, you can U-turn your mind to further embrace impermanence. You can move forward with dedication and energy toward your purpose and path, with appreciation for the supportive conditions of your life right now, including gratitude for your loved ones who have come and gone.

We have day. We have night. We have life. We have death. Maybe I'm a day person. I like the light. But I must go through the night, too. If I accept night, sleep, darkness, then I'm ready for it when it comes. Everything is impermanent. Everything is changing except change. You need to know, really know, that your life is impermanent. You will die. You could think about this for a few minutes each day as medicine for your mind.

Suffering of Samsara

It sounds dramatic—the suffering of samsara. It also sounds distant—someone is suffering over there in samsara. But we are in samsara. And we are suffering. First of all, what is samsara? Samsara is the wheel of life. The best example is the hamster wheel. The hamster is running and running. Why? Because that's what you do in the wheel. The hamster is like business people, running all day because they are busy. But we are all business people because we are all busy people. Whether we are in business or not, our business is busy-ness. We are constantly running in various systems of culture, tradition, society, education, religion as well as the internal mental states conditioned by these systems—toxic attachment, anger, jealousy, pride, arrogance, and so on. Having been conditioned, we keep the conditioning going. While we are running in the wheel, we are simultaneously constructing it for ourselves and others. So we are running in the cycle of systems that is samsara. This running is what we think of as living. This running is how we know we are alive.

What is the problem with this kind of life? What is the suffering? Make a list right now of your problems, your basic life problems. Maybe you have married-people problems. Maybe you have single-people problems. Maybe you have people-with-kids problems. Maybe you have people-without-kids problems. Maybe you have work problems. Maybe you have no-work problems. Maybe you have money problems. Maybe you have no-money problems. Maybe you have sex problems. Maybe you have no-sex problems. Maybe you have exercise problems. Maybe you have no-exercise problems. Some may say no no—don't think about problems. Think only positive thoughts, especially in spirituality. But spirituality is about your real life. And the preliminary practice is about getting real about your real life. Life is full of problems, conflicts, misunderstandings, and failures. Even if we want to think of things only happening this good way or that good way, life goes its own way. Or maybe things seem good right now, but there is always the potential for pain and problems. Also, there are problems all around us, even if they don't seem like our problems. And we share collective problems, like political problems and climate problems. But, for now, look at your problems. It's not like we don't have problems if we practice spirituality. Talk of bliss is coming, but we have to start in real life with our problems. Anything can happen, even to so-called spiritual people.

There was a famous nun in India. She was a princess from a rich family who became a nun. Then she got sick with leprosy. It got so bad that she lost her fingers. Nobody wanted to come close to her; even her spiritual community kicked her out. So she made her own journey. Later, she said that time in her life, while suffering terribly on her own, was when she really found her true inner spiritual path—because in her own suffering, she could better understand the suffering of others. A feeling of compassion naturally arose in her, and she wanted to take the pain of others. She wanted to take on their sicknesses so they could be cured. She fasted and did a mantra practice focused on compassion. She actually self-healed and was completely cured. She said the most difficult part of her life was the best part of her spiritual journey. She U-turned from wrong view to right view.

So think very clearly about your problems and see how you are surrounded by others with their problems. You do not need to judge your problems, and you definitely do not need to judge others' problems. It is very normal to have physical problems and emotional problems and mental problems and all kinds of problems. This is the nature of life in the wheel of samsara, with all its conditioning in wrong view. By paying attention to the reality of samsara, maybe you will begin to have the nun's U-turn thought of compassion—wanting to put an end to this suffering for others and yourself. See if right view begins to dawn. You could think about this for a few minutes each day as medicine for your mind.

Karma—Cause and Effect

Traditionally, karma—cause and effect—is taught before the suffering of samsara. But, sometimes, it makes sense to teach it afterward. Because now we get to think carefully about why we are suffering in samsara. Why are we continuing to run in this wheel of conditioning? Why are we repeating thoughts, words, and actions that cause pain for ourselves and others? What is the wrong view fueling this cyclical situation?

Think again about your list of problems. Every single one of your problems has a primary cause and probably many secondary causes. The preliminary practice is about building awareness of our own problems and their causes. Though life is complex, we can break down the process of our experiences, including our problems. This analysis is a U-turn from ignorance to insight. It is right view. Start with something basic. If you did something good yesterday, maybe today you are relaxed and happy. It's like a wave from yesterday's good action to today's relaxation and happiness. Karma means action. Our mental and physical states are all karmic waves. If we are sad, there's a reason why we are sad. If we are happy, there's a reason why we are happy. Anything can happen in your mind and body and life, but there is always a reason. Sometimes you don't see the reason, but it doesn't mean there is no reason. If you create good causes and conditions in your mind and body and life, you will receive good things in your mind and body and life. Karma is universal justice; nobody can run away from cause and effect.

But here is the big point about karma—the primary cause of all of your problems is your response to life. Even when it seems like the cause of your problems is something external, the real issue is how you respond to these external factors. How do you respond to personal situations, family situations, work situations, community situations, national situations, global situations? In productive, creative, harmonizing, openhearted ways? In unproductive, divisive, hostile, self-centered ways? On the spiritual path, it is imperative to examine how we are causing our own problems. We like to blame others for our problems—complaining about the boss, partner, kids, friends, neighbors, strangers, government, environment. But this is wrong view. The real problem is that we don't know how to manage our own minds and lives. We don't know how to manage our anger. We don't know how to manage our laziness. We don't know how to manage our desire. We don't know how to manage our loneliness. We are confused, and we don't know we are confused. We must think carefully—why am I angry today, why was I angry yesterday, why was I angry the day before yesterday, why am I angry every day? Did you know you are angry every day? Don't deny it. You are angry every day for different reasons. Anger is an organic human emotion. You don't need to feel bad about anger or jealousy or any other toxic emotion. Nor do you need to feel under its power. This little anger comes up like a bubble, but it has a cause. If you are angry, if you are unhappy mentally, if you have health issues, ask yourself why—there are reasons in your own mind and life.

If you are unable to think about how and why you cause your problems, you are not practicing spirituality. The preliminary practice invites you to U-turn from blaming others to taking responsibility for your emotions and choices. This is right view. You must examine how much you are conditioned in your reactions to personal, familial, professional, national, and global situations. Samsara seems like an unstoppable wheel, but it is only moving because of karma—cause and effect. Your reactions—toxic thoughts, emotions, words, and actions—are what spin the wheel of suffering for yourself and others. Of course, in the Buddhist teachings, this wheel does not stop spinning after this life. We spin in the wheel from life to life. Maybe the mindstream runs in the body of a hamster in this life, then flies as a bird in the next life, then slithers as a snake in the next life, then hustles as a business person in the next life. It is all the same cycle of conditioned and repetitive responses.

Through spiritual practice, you can find your unconditioned nature, free of mental poisons and toxins. At that level, it is not that you do not care about what happens, but what happens is not influencing you or affecting you in the ways that it always has. You are free of habitual karmic waves—free to act with loving kindness, compassion, joy, and equanimity instead of reacting with ignorance, desire, anger, jealousy, and pride. What might be underneath all of your cyclical conditioning? Think about the nun with leprosy—her naturally arising compassion for others and joy in her journey. That potential exists in us all. But, for now, we are very much conditioned. You can U-turn from being conditioned to being unconditioned, from wrong view to right view, by repeatedly looking at how you are causing your problems. You could think about this for a few minutes each day as medicine for your mind.

Once we begin taking the medicine of the Four U-Turn Thoughts, then we know why we practice spirituality. We are not using spirituality to bypass our real lives and emotions and problems. Rather we are looking directly at our lives—the value of our lives, the impermanence of our lives, the suffering of our lives, and the causes for that suffering. We have a very precise reason to practice. We do not want to get stuck in the cycle of repeatedly bringing pain and suffering to ourselves and others. Then spiritual practice becomes logical and serious. Thinking about these things for a few minutes each day can turn the mind toward right view, which displays in right thought, right speech, and right action. Again, the common Ngöndro contributes to a strong spiritual childhood, from which we can grow into mature spiritual practitioners. This is the same journey the Buddha took—into reality and right view. So, now, we will turn to his teaching on the Four Noble Truths, another initial medicine that invites us into a lifetime of healing and balance.

THE FOUR NOBLE TRUTHS

The Four Noble Truths is a basic medical model.

Here is an example:

1. You have a chronic headache.
2. There is a cause of this headache.
3. There is a cessation of this headache.
4. There is a path leading to this cessation.

To employ this medical model, you would examine your headache, such as when and how it arises. Based on your examination, you would determine the cause of your headache—maybe stress, dehydration, or too much alcohol or sugar. Now knowing the cause, you would know how to end this headache and prevent future headaches. Then, based on your diagnosis, you would cut back on stress or increase water intake or cool it with the alcohol or sugar. This is a simple and methodical way to heal oneself.

Here are the Four Noble Truths:

1. Life is suffering.
2. There is a cause of this suffering.
3. There is a cessation of this suffering.
4. There is a path leading to this cessation.

To employ this medical model, you would examine your suffering, such as when and how it arises. Based on your examination, you would determine the cause of your suffering. Now knowing the cause, you would know how to end this suffering and prevent future suffering. Then, based on your diagnosis, you would take the medicine that addresses this cause. This is a simple and methodical way to heal oneself.

Indeed, this medical model is the prescription the Buddha has written for us all to free ourselves from suffering. Maybe you are noticing the difference between the headache example and the Four Noble Truths above—the details of the cause and the path are left out of the description of the Four Noble Truths. That's because it would spoil the story to state the solution at the start! Also, the Buddha didn't know the cause of suffering at the start of his journey. He went looking for suffering's cause and solution, and his path is applicable to us all.

Truth #1—Life is Suffering

Again with the suffering? First it dominates the Four U-Turn Thoughts, and now it starts off the Four Noble Truths. All this talk of suffering is why Buddhists have a bad reputation for being downers. Many religious traditions talk about divine power, love and light, miraculous healing, benevolent universe, high vibrations. Popular spirituality promotes manifesting positive things with positive thoughts. And, these days, there is great interest in positive psychology and positive mindsets. That is all fine. But we also have to know the reality of life. Sometimes when we only talk about good things, it is like an escape. If you want good health, you often need to know the specifics of the disease so you can determine the cure and course of treatment. If our language is up in the sky, we are not grounded. Then, when we experience pain and suffering, we feel confused and even betrayed by our relentlessly positive spiritual path. Buddhism starts on the ground with ordinary life—your problems and complaints and mental issues.

The Buddha Shakyamuni, the historical Buddha of our time, went looking for a solution to basic suffering—old age, sickness, death, and rebirth. It does not get more grounded than that. He undertook this journey because he had been shielded from reality. He was a great prince with everything a young boy can have. He was known for his art and study and sport. Yet he was still internally unhappy and dissatisfied. He wanted to leave the royal palace and travel, but his father forbade him from any exploration. His father wanted to create the illusion that royal life was perfect, his family was perfect, there was no pain, and there were no problems. Though it is an extreme example, we all share this situation. We are all raised in an enclosed palace as bonsai within a cozy pot of mental conditioning. Yet we are dissatisfied. We suspect there is more to know and see; we want to taste the freedom of the forest. However, we are prevented from this exploration by conditioned circumstances for some of us and by conditioned thoughts for all of us, including those spiritual thoughts that create a positivity palace in our minds.

Seeking truth, the Buddha snuck out of his conditioned palatial circumstances four times in four different directions, and he witnessed the four basic human sufferings—old age, sickness, death, rebirth. Then the Buddha had a question: Is there any solution for this suffering? Despite being well educated, the Buddha had been denied spiritual teachings because his father did not want anything to threaten the status quo of their picture-perfect existence. We can understand a father's love for his son, including having his heart set on his boy following in his footsteps as the next king. Again, many of us have been restricted by our conditioned social/cultural/familial paths, and all of us have been restricted by our conditioned neural pathways. But the Buddha desperately wanted to find an antidote for these sufferings; he was more interested in helping humanity than becoming a king. So he gave up his royal palace and family, and he escaped to explore spirituality with the hope of benefiting beings. With vigor, he dove into the ascetic spiritual practices of the time, and he nearly died. Then he was given a bit of rice milk, regained his strength, found a Bodhi tree, and made a promise—until I find the inner solution to suffering, I will not stand up from my meditation. His meditation lasted six years. Most of us go on retreat and meditate for a few sessions each day, maybe have chitchat with friends over meals. This was not that. He sat in meditation for six years. He did not get up. He made the ultimate inner journey into the human mind. He saw the different layers and angles of the human mind, all the corners and nooks and crannies.

In so doing, he discovered that humans have 84,000 possible mental problems. How many mental problems do you think you have? Maybe one or two or five? Not so many compared to 84,000. Sometimes a mental problem can seem so big, but it is just one. We can have 84,000. All of these mental problems comprise our disease of suffering.

The Buddha broke down the disease of suffering into eight categories—the four he initially wanted to heal and four more:

- Old age

- Sickness

- Death

- Rebirth

- Suffering of meeting. This is encountering something you don't like. It could be a person you don't like, a problem you don't like, a situation you don't like, an experience you don't like. Things like that.

- Suffering of separation. This is being separated from something you do like. It could be family or friends or partners that you part from through death or distance or dispute, satisfying work that is over, something you created and lost, a beautiful object that is now gone, a pleasant experience or time that has passed. Things like that.

- Suffering of not finding what you want. This is never finding what you are looking for in life. It could be the perfect partner, inspiring work, a beautiful home, an ideal meditation situation, an object of desire, an experience of pleasure. Things like that.

- Suffering in body and mind. This is never being satisfied with your body. You think you are too small, too big, too old, too young, too ugly, too pretty, too tall, too short. There is always something wrong with your body. It also includes never being satisfied with your mind. You have all these feelings and worries, and you don't know why you're not happy. Things like that.

He further expounded upon the disease of suffering with three types of suffering that pervade the eight categories:

- Suffering of suffering. Suffering causes us pain. And we add layers of suffering to any suffering. This can be called the second arrow. You have a painful physical or mental experience (first arrow), and then you have a painful thought or feeling about that pain (second arrow). You have a toothache (first arrow), and you don't like having a toothache (second arrow). You are angry (first arrow), and you are judging yourself for being angry (second arrow). You are aging (first arrow), and you have sadness about being older (second arrow). You add a second layer, maybe even more, to the initial suffering.

- Changing suffering. In the beginning, you thought something was good, but then it transformed into suffering. The classic example is love dramas. Those first days or months or even years we are in love, we lose our head; it is so good, oh love, love, love. There is joy and happiness. But we all know how this movie ends. That love transforms into one of the most painful sufferings, as breakups or death or something pulls you and your lover apart. Another example could be our relentlessly positive spiritual path where everything is good and uplifted and magical at the start; but then things go sideways in our lives, and our positive thinking isn't working, and we judge ourselves or our spirituality or our teachers.

- All-pervasive suffering. Suffering is everywhere in our lives. You always have a problem. Wherever you go, there's a problem. Whenever you look at the news, there's a problem. Whoever you meet, they have a problem. Or maybe you don't have a problem, but somebody has a problem with you. There is no end to our problems.

Truth #2—There is a Cause of this Suffering

So here we are with 84,000 mental problems falling into these various categories and types of suffering. One would think the cause of all this suffering would be very complicated, needing to be expounded upon with lists and subsections as well. That is not the case. There is a single cause of your suffering—it is you. It is the concept of you. It is the toxic, ignorant notion that you exist as an independent entity to star in the show of your success and your suffering. This is the ultimate wrong view.

In reality, when you take the time and find the courage to explore your mind and life, you see that everything, including you, is created by countless causes and conditions coming together in interdependence. Therefore, while we need to have names for things, these things do not have static, solid, inherent existence. Everything is fluid and dynamic and in relationship with everything else. This is called emptiness—as in, empty of a separate self but full of interconnection. Emptiness sounds cool. We like to talk about it. We like to talk about the emptiness of all phenomena—a house, the ocean, any political situation. It feels freeing to see the interconnectivity and complexity of it all. We can get kind of high on the theory of emptiness. We feel smart and special when we wax philosophical about not being able to grasp the solidity of a "tree" or even land in the "present."

However, our excitement about emptiness may fade when we truly contemplate what this means about ourselves—and our concept of a self. When you examine how interdependent causes and conditions continually come together to create ever-changing you, you see that there is no star-of-the-show you. There is no self in the way we think of a self—this can be called selflessness. When we encounter this teaching, we'll still get a little high on the theory of emptiness and make jokes as if we accept selflessness. But to come down from the theory of emptiness and land in the reality of selflessness, you must reckon with the realization that the concept of you is your only problem. In truth, there is no static, solid, inherent you that exists to experience all of this success or suffering. What you interpret as your life—with all its dramas including your extraordinary gifts and your precious specialness and your annoying neighbor and your unreasonable ex and your death and rebirth—is a conceptual activity. It is a fabrication. This self that you cherish, protect, and defend, much to the suffering of yourself and others, is only a conditioned habit of mind, speech, and body.

To put it another way: The cause of your headache is thinking you have a head. You don't.

In your heart, you know this. As evidence, you can create your story of self many different ways each day, and you do depending on things as minor as whether you pooped this morning and are feeling good or whether you didn't poop and are feeling bad. The ignorance of believing in a story of self—and sticking to it—is the original mental toxin. All of our toxins, our 84,000 mental problems, our eight categories and three types of suffering, stem from such ignorance. Our true nature is free from self, free from I. Again, the theory sounds great. If you don't have a head, you can't have a headache. But meditating on the emptiness of self and other, really absorbing this, is the most difficult challenge of our lives because we are so deeply conditioned to believe in the concept of me and you, subject and object, as solid and separate entities. In reality, you are completely free from all of the stories and dramas and concepts of self and other as well as all of the suffering that ensues from that toxic, dualistic ignorance.

You can think of your conditioning of self as contracting. Maybe you have had an experience of an expanded state, where you forgot yourself—during creative flow, the athletic zone, incredible sex, a fantastic massage, a drug-induced trip. Being free of self, you felt easy and relaxed and open. It was so easy and relaxed and open that it was hard to trust the experience. You thought you weren't allowed to stay there or you didn't know how. You reflexively remembered I, and that contraction felt comfortable, like a security blanket. So you shrank back into I—reinvesting in the dramas of self, which reify this experience of I. I'm this; I'm that. The more you build the force of I—through thoughts of self, stories of self, actions promoting self—the more you contract and collect problems. You have been doing this for your entire life—many lives say the Buddhists. We are all conditioned to construct the self, and we are conditioning each other to do the same. Through our thoughts, speech, and actions, we encourage each other's toxic delusion of dualism all the time.

Let's imagine this contraction in terms of our elemental makeup. Let's say, originally, you are a crystal clear drop of water. Then, because of ignorance, you contract into an icicle. Then, because of conditioning, you roll like a snowball for years upon years, lives upon lives, becoming a glacier of self with all of your stories. Or let's say, originally, you are a gentle breeze. Then, because of ignorance, you contract into a funnel cloud. Then, because of conditioning, you pick up dust and debris for years upon years, lives upon lives, becoming a cyclone of self with all of your stories. Or let's say, originally, you are a spark of light. Then, because of ignorance, you contract into a flame. Then, because of conditioning, you pick up kindling and brush for years upon years, lives upon lives, becoming an inferno of self with all of your stories.

We think we have problems and struggles because of external conditions. But the problem is that we don't realize our true inner nature. We say it's important to be myself—but we are mostly this conditioned and superficial self. Because of ignorance, you don't even know what you are. And, until you do, you are the source of your own suffering. All suffering has a cause—the ignorance of self. If you know the cause clearly, then you can prevent the disease. At the end, you are the doctor and the patient. You are not the victim of suffering. As the Buddha showed us, you can heal yourself. This is right view.

Truth #3—There is a Cessation of this Suffering

Once you realize your inner nature of emptiness, you are free from conditions. If you master your mind, you master your energy and body. Once you master yourself, you master everything. You can be clear, comfortable, and compassionate in any situation—any situation.

It is the ultimate understatement to say that it was not easy for the Buddha to reach this realization of emptiness. You have probably sat in meditation. You know what the mind does. You know how self tries to keep the stories going. So, too, the Buddha was attacked by the maras, or demons. First, the maras tried anger and aggression, shooting arrows and throwing swords and spears. Then, the maras' desirable daughters arrived, all sexy and inviting. Again, you have probably sat in meditation; you know what happens. The maras taunted him saying, "You are a mess; you are not enlightened." Then the Buddha said, "I have my witness to my enlightenment; it is the Mother Earth." And he touched the Mother Earth. With that, the maras' weapons became flowers. With that, the maras' daughters became flowers. With that, the Buddha was free from external conditions.

The moment he was enlightened, he became the Buddha, the awakened one. He woke up from ignorance, the root cause of all suffering. He was completely clear. His wisdom was completely developed. He had found something profound and peaceful, free from fabrications, the infinite clear light, without creators or creation process, not made in China or India or Tibet or by the Buddha—it was just there. Like nectar, it heals all. It transforms negative into positive. It transforms poison into medicine. It transforms demons into buddhas. He found the Dharma, the truth. He was speechless. And he wondered if people would even understand him if he did speak. He stayed in the forest for seven weeks. Then the request came from disciples and invisible gods to teach, and he taught the Four Noble Truths. He came out of six years of deep meditation, now awakened, and spoke about the answers to his own questions.

The Buddha found that we all have Buddha Nature. This is also called rigpa, the primordial state of mind. It is also called yeshe, pristine consciousness. It is the highest consciousness, completely awakened, the ultimate nature of the human mind. It is free of pain and suffering. It is free of all mental confusions and mental toxins. It is free of self.

Notice in the Buddha's story that the maras taunted him by saying that he was not enlightened as they sent him all manner of distractions. This is what our ignorant stories of self do. They feed us desire, anger, pride, jealousy, and so on. They do this all day; they do this in our dreams. We see it more when we meditate because we are looking at the mind. But, like the Buddha, we are also already awakened. Our Buddha Nature is within—uncreated, luminous, and healing. This is true for every single being. Welcome to the ultimate right view.

Truth #4—There is a Path Leading to this Cessation

The Buddha continued to teach and prescribe for his students a path to reach this state of awakening or enlightenment. And so, the process of waking up came to be known as Buddhism. There are debates about whether Buddhism is religion, philosophy, science, or psychology. In general, we need to respect everyone and relax about defining Buddhism. The way you enter this path is up to you, your culture, and your tradition. Some people find peace and joy with religion, so Buddhism manifests as religion for them. For philosophers, Buddhism manifests as philosophy. The scientists see Buddhism aligns with science. The psychologists think of Buddhism as psychology. I'm a Sowa Rigpa doctor, so the psychological approach makes sense for me. I see Buddhism as the antidote to our mental toxins, which heals our energetic and physical toxins as well. This means that all of your problems can be cured, according to the Buddha. Your suffering can completely cease.

The Tibetan words for Buddhism describe it as an inner science. Inner science means inner awareness—of your physical body, energetic body, and mind. This path covers everything about us. And the more we understand ourselves, the more we understand others. Once we understand the inner dimension, we understand the outer dimension. Inner and outer are always connected and related. As we wake up, we understand that nothing is separate. Indeed, through this inner science, we realize the right view of nondualism and display this wisdom through right thought, right speech, and right action. All of which promote what is known as the Four Immeasurables—loving kindness, compassion, joy, and equanimity—which we can offer in any situation.

One of the most skillful aspects of the Buddha's medicine, or the Buddhist path, is its variety of methods. The Buddha saw that we have potentially 84,000 mental problems. Well, don't worry, because he found 84,000 solutions. Each poison has a medicine. The Buddha taught different teachings for different people—we like different foods, we have different skills, we get different teachings. Maybe your medicine looks like religion to you; maybe my medicine looks like psychology to me. No matter which antidote you need, this array of medicines has developed into two main styles of inner science—sutra and tantra. In simple terms, sutra involves renunciation and tantra involves transformation. With sutra, you renounce your worldly life for a spiritual life. With tantra, you remain in your worldly life and skillfully transform it into spirituality.

In this time and place, most people seem to gravitate toward tantra over sutra. It's not hard to see why. We hear that sutra is the path of renunciation and tantra is the path of transformation. Without knowing exactly what that means, most of us would rather transform than renounce. In a world dominated by consumer capitalism, giving up things is not our forte. We hear that sutra is the moon, and tantra is the sun. Compared to the moonlight, the sunlight is stronger. Meaning, on the sutra path, enlightenment can take many lifetimes; on the tantra path, we can get enlightened in one lifetime. And most of us would rather get enlightened in this lifetime under the bright sun. We hear that sutra is the root and tantra is the fruit. And most of us would rather eat the fruit than the root. So, as busy and lazy and even greedy people, tantra seems like the natural choice.

Perhaps a more charitable view of why we gravitate toward tantra has to do with the psychological needs of this time. The two paths have a different emphasis at the start. The sutra path begins with talk of suffering because our lives are full of problems. Through sutra teachings and practices, we cease suffering by realizing emptiness, especially of the self. With that realization of emptiness, and complete release of self-attachment, we experience the bliss of Buddha Nature. However, the tantra path begins with talk of bliss rather than suffering. In tantra, we say, "We were all born with bliss. We all live with bliss. We all die with bliss." The problem is that we don't experience bliss because mental poisons dominate our mind, causing us mental, energetic, and physical suffering. Through tantric teachings and practices, we reconnect with our inherent bliss and remember our Buddha Nature, which also results in our release of self-attachment and thus cessation of suffering. To put it in more psychological terms, the opposite of stress and suffering is not only the absence of stress and suffering but also the presence of joy and bliss. Maybe, in this time and place, we hear too much about stress and suffering already. Maybe it helps us to hear more about joy and bliss from the start. So maybe that is why we naturally gravitate toward tantra these days.

That said, thinking we are choosing between two paths is misguided. They are really two sides of the same hand. Tibetan Buddhism actually finds the middle way of sutra and tantra. Both schools are woven into the practice path. That way, we don't have to choose or have extreme views. We do not need to be concerned about which style we practice, and we definitely do not need to be concerned about which style others practice. To each their own. Let's look briefly at both styles of practice to better understand where Yuthok's heart-essence teachings fit.

Again, sutra is characterized as the path of renunciation. Hearing that, we mostly think about external renunciation—such as monastics giving up so-called worldly activities like sex and family life, hair and outfits, jobs and alcohol. However, true renunciation is a mental state. You could physically renounce everything under the sun and still be plagued by thoughts of craving, anger, pride, and jealousy. The key point of renunciation is to release attachment to the self and its ensuing mental poisons.

Thus, sutra practices go after the self, exposing it as the sham it is. Sutra practitioners do Shamatha and Vipassana meditation. Of course, tantra practitioners can do these meditations as well, but they are sutra styled. Shamatha is calm abiding meditation, and there are many different forms of this. Essentially, you learn how to let the mind become still, quiet, and peaceful. With lots of practice, your mind ceases to stir up stories of self; instead, your mind rests in the present moment.

If you can maintain calm abiding for at least sixty minutes, you have a stable base of Shamatha. It can take many years of very hard training to accomplish this, which can be especially difficult for laypeople with jobs and families and full schedules. Professional Shamatha practitioners might reside in mountain caves and monasteries, and they stay in calm abiding for hours or days, even always. Today, there is a lot of superficial Shamatha, but deep Shamatha is steady and profound. Once you have a stable Shamatha foundation of an hour, you can try Vipassana meditation where you look at your mind. This is also known as analytical meditation or insight meditation. Shamatha is turning on the light, and Vipassana is seeing clearly in the room. If the light is turning on and off, you can't get a clear look around the room. But once that light is on, you can see clearly how your thoughts and feelings are empty in nature. You can see clearly the emptiness of self and the ignorance of self-other, or subject-object, dualism. Though these practices require many years of training, the reward is liberation. You explore mind, you explore self, and you can realize emptiness. With this realization, Buddha Nature dawns, as it did for the Buddha who also engaged in these practices.

Sutra also helps us see that there is freedom in discipline—specifically, the discipline in not indulging in the notion of a self with its traumas and dramas. External renunciation is a tool to support the internal renunciation of self-attachment. For some practitioners, external renunciation may feel forced at first. However, over time, they lose interest in everything except the sweet bliss of Buddha Nature and the compassionate activity it inspires, including the fierce compassion of boundary setting. So their seemingly rigid external renunciation actually feels very natural and easy. For some, the internal renunciation of self may come first, freeing them from any desire to participate in activities that stir up a sense of self-attachment—worldly activities that may be culturally normalized but are not cultivating balance, health, or sanity. Whatever order they arise, internal and external renunciation are aligned. And, for these practitioners, it is delicious to lose all taste for mental poisons and whatever cooks them up. Relaxing into renunciation, sutra practitioners can fully focus on being of benefit to beings through loving kindness, compassion, joy, and equanimity.

As the path of transformation, tantra takes a different approach.

Rather than renounce the self straightaway, the practices use the self to transform the self. The practices leverage our habitual self-fascination to mentally recreate ourselves as buddhas and deities and then attune our body, speech, and mind to our inherent Buddha Nature and bliss. Essentially, the practices transmute your mental poisons into your medicine. As such, there are different tantras for different toxins as well as different lifestyles and different times. Indeed, the tantric practices we will explore in this book arise from a specific tantra for this time in humanity and existence. Without going into an extensive description, there was once a time when beings had bodies made of light, they ate only nectar, they were flying instead of walking, they didn't have sexes, and they felt great satisfaction and joy just looking at each other. That may sound improbable or fanciful, but you remember it somewhere in your being. Surely, you have experienced a shiver of pleasure at simply the sight of your new lover or a sense of satiety from soaking in a sunset. Over time, beings have become denser. We have lost bodies of light and flight; we have lost the capacity for joy just through sight. In this time, our human sensory experience is very intense. We are embodied in fleshy bodies. We need to eat solid food. We display sexes and genders. We have carnal desires that we fulfill through contact and intercourse and aggression. Essentially, we have a world plagued by craving and fighting. It is what it is. And it requires a specific tantra.

In fact, there are a few different tantras for this time of incarnation. The tantra taught in this lineage, and many of today's spiritual lineages, is an Anuttarayoga tantra. This tantra teaches a process of working internally that makes no demands of external renunciation. You can eat meat, drink alcohol, have sex, have a family, have a job, grow your hair, and wear whatever. These days, this lack of external rules is often misinterpreted as breaking rules for the hell of it. When actually, tantra shares a basic code of ethical conduct with sutra—namely, abandoning the ten wrong actions of body, speech, and mind (killing, stealing, sexual misconduct, lying, idle and harsh and divisive speech, covetousness/greediness, ill-will, and wrong view). In reality, this tantra was designed for people who were unable to meet the sutra standards of renunciation or other tantras' requirements of purity around behavior, hygiene, and diet. Honestly, it was designed for people who didn't have a doorway into monasticism or didn't have a lot of resources or didn't have much choice about breaking rules for survival—people who needed to hustle for work, who needed to sell their bodies to eat, who needed to fight to stay safe, who needed to drink alcohol to fit into culture. Anuttarayoga tantra is designed to be street style, doing the basics without getting hung up on notions of good and bad that could disqualify people from being seen as spiritual practitioners or seeing themselves as spiritual practitioners. Maybe right now some of us need to be street style to survive. Or maybe some of us have minds and lives so tightly bound by bonsai pots that certain kinds of renunciation seem impossible or unappealing. Or maybe some of us find contemporary spirituality's one-note wellness, homogeneous fashion sense, fancy food, and corporate mind-body trends are out of reach monetarily or out of step culturally or out of alignment personally. Whatever the case, Anuttarayoga tantra frees us from rejecting or refusing any aspect of life, as it was created for those without the privilege to be picky about their lifestyles. So, setting external rules aside, we work with our internal energies. After all, who cares about self-appearance when you are filled with bliss. Even better, who cares about others' appearances when you know we all possess Buddha Nature.

So this is where we start on the tantric path—knowing that every single being possesses the seed of Buddha Nature. These practices do not add anything; they reveal what is already there. The practices of this tantra fall within two main categories—creation stage and completion stage. Though often people practicing these practices may not even know this, these two stages are designed according to time—past and future. We have problems of the past, and we have problems of the future. We have fear of the past, and we have fear of the future. Sometimes, we get stuck in the past—all of our problems come from memories, from childhood until now. So, with creation stage, we go back to the moment we were conceived and recreate ourselves from then to here and now. Sometimes, we get stuck in the future—all of our problems are projections, worries, and possible sorrows about getting old, getting sick, and dying. So, with completion stage, we journey into our future, to our death, when our elements will dissolve into the clear light. That said, for the most part, these practices do not name that we are essentially working with our past conception and future death. Tantra is chill like that. Instead, through visualization, breathing, mantra, and movement, you clear your mental toxins and blah blahs about the past and future.

With creation stage practices, you transform toxins to medicines by visualizing yourself as a buddha or deity. This is an endeavor in both imagination and recognition. You know you are not expressing the body, speech, and mind of a buddha right now, but you know you can express the body, speech, and mind of a buddha because you have the seed of Buddha Nature. So, through visualization, you are recreating yourself into what you truly are—a buddha. Creation stage is also called generation stage. You are regenerating yourself into whatever type of buddha resonates for you. Maybe you have a lot of anger, so you want to be a warrior buddha holding weapons symbolizing compassion instead of violence. Maybe you have a lot of desire, so you want to be a sexy buddha wearing jewels symbolizing wisdom instead of attachment. Depending on what toxins you have and teachings you receive, there are countless deities and buddhas to experience through creation stage. Again, every poison has a medicine. We have peaceful medicines, wrathful medicines, joyful medicines. Or maybe you need medicines of equilibrium. Maybe you are female-bodied in this life but want to generate as a male-bodied buddha to balance your energy. Maybe you are male-bodied this life but want to generate as a female-bodied buddha to balance your energy. Maybe you are nonbinary this life and want to generate as a union of buddhas to support your energy in a dualistic culture that may not support your nondual being. Maybe you are subdued this life and want to generate as bold. Maybe you are bold this life and want to generate as subdued. Creation stage can be personalized according to your psychology, energy, and mentality. Your teachers can help you understand and access the medicines of buddhas and deities that fit your needs. They may even suggest you generate as something surprising—calling forth your awakened internal expression that they can see but you may not yet.

Once you have recreated your body as a buddha, your creation continues. You can recite the mantra of the buddha that you are practicing, thus aligning your body and your speech-energy in this recreation. Then, with your mind, you visualize or imagine or feel yourself radiating light as the buddha you are. You radiate light in all directions as an offering to all of the buddhas and deities. Then you receive light back from them as a blessing and support. Then you radiate light again to bless and support all sentient beings. And that's when the real magic happens—because the brilliance of creation stage practice is that it does not stop with you. Remember that every sentient being possesses the seed of Buddha Nature. So, as you radiate light to bless and support all sentient beings, they also recreate into the buddhas they truly are. During this practice, we change our perception into pure view, seeing all sentient beings, from insects to animals to our next-door neighbors, as buddhas. This means that as we recreate ourselves, we recreate the whole universe. When you say, "I" this I is the center of your universe. If you change your understanding of I, you will change your understanding of literally everything. It is a huge psychological and beneficial shift.

However, though you are recreating as the blissful buddha you actually are, creation stage is not at all about the denial of human life. In Anuttarayoga tantra, you might recreate as deities and buddhas holding skull cups filled with blood, wearing necklaces of skulls, draped in animal skins, even having animal heads. It can get a little wild. The other tantras of this time don't talk about things like death, blood, and so on. Everything is clean in those tantras. This is often the case in our human life, too. We want to have a nice bowl and a proper cup. We want to drink delicious tea. If we want everything to be clean and pretty for us, we might be shocked by some of the images in Anuttarayoga tantra. But, in our human life, we might not realize that in order to get our precious shiitake-mushroom tea, the farmers killed thousands of insects to protect and harvest the mushrooms. That cup of tea is actually a cup of blood. Or maybe in our human life we want to dress ourselves in pretty outfits and emotions, while we deny our anger, lust, jealousy, pride, and so on. But, in Anuttarayoga tantra, we are now transforming our toxins into medicines. So we harness the all-consuming experience of emotions into being wrathful, sensual, and powerful buddhas. Then we actually feel the organically wise and compassionate energetic nature of our so-called poisons. Ultimately, we need to understand the essence of emotions and pain and life and death. We need to break free from our pretty pots of conditioning to see what is really going on here. Otherwise, we can use spirituality, and its supposed purity and goodness, as another form of escapism. This does not mean that we should try to do things that are harmful and selfish in order to break conditioning. Remember that the root of sutra undergirds the fruit of tantra, and they both include non-harming as part of compassionate action. All of this wild and shocking imagery simply helps us see the truths of this precious human life: One, it is impossible to exist anywhere in the cycle of samsara without experiencing and inflicting suffering. Two, you have the power to break the cycle of pain, right here and right now.

Creation stage leads to completion stage. Once you have recreated as a buddha, you dive into the inner dimension of your body, speech-energy, and mind. As we will discuss, there are a variety of completion stage practices. Again, there are medicines for all the toxins. Generally speaking, with completion stage practice, we work with a system of energetic channels within the body. Then our breathing, thinking, moving, sleeping, dreaming, love making (with self or other), and even dying become opportunities to transform our confusion into wisdom. These practices allow us to experience our inherent bliss and Buddha Nature directly. We lose attachment to the self, as we now know it, because we come to know ourselves, and everyone else, as a buddha. We see that we do not need to look elsewhere for anything. Everything is complete internally. Everything you need to wake up is within you.

With creation and completion stage practices, you realize that you can generate and dissolve in any way, shape, or form that you would like. Life reveals itself to be the dynamic play of energy and elements. You can experience the reality of selflessness—feeling the fullness and expansiveness of generating and dissolving, again and again, as you take all kinds of forms in this life and beyond.

Tantra and sutra can both bring us to realization. In fact, tantra's creation and completion stage practices are not unlike sutra's Shamatha and Vipassana practices. With creation stage, you calm your mind by concentrating on your visualization. With completion stage, you see your mind as it truly is—awake. The difference is that results can happen more quickly through tantra than sutra. Again, it is said that tantra can liberate you in a single lifetime. As mentioned, Tibetan Buddhism uses a combination of sutra and tantra. Most of the Tibetan monks and nuns are ordained in a sutra way. They keep all of their external renunciation, and internally they practice tantra. There is no contradiction between the two. My teachers are monks and nuns. My primary teacher of Buddhism, also known as a root guru, was a fully ordained nun. My root guru for the Yuthok Nyingthig was a fully ordained monk. Again, I took the path of the ngakpa—non-monastic, non-celibate yogi—because my medicine involves having my inner and outer expression match, having it all be the natural style of Anuttarayoga tantra.

The Yuthok Nyingthig, which we will dive into in the next chapter, is an Anuttarayoga tantra. It was designed for this time, and I have found it to be a perfect fit. These days, in addition to being busy and lazy, most of us have distracted and critical minds. Sutra texts have a lot of theory and not much explanation, and they can be kind of boring. Sutra meditations can also be kind of boring. I struggled with them when I was young. Tantra has many exciting meditations and visualizations. It also gives us many explanations and has many practices. Sutra says, "You can eat rice or spaghetti, that's it." Tantra says, "There's salad, tofu, fish, beans, lasagna, steak, cake, pie." There are many dishes. We can choose the practices that are more effective for us. Also, we are not living in a time and place that supports renunciation, let alone monasticism. Further, most Westerners tend to encounter Dharma later in their lives. Maybe you are a little older and already have a nice place, a stable job, and a family. With tantra, you do not need to avoid or abandon what you have. You can incorporate your entire life into the path. As we will discuss, you can visualize offering your good fortune over and over again to the buddhas. So you don't need to change much. You just need to know the practice and do the practice. Whatever you have in your life can become part of your spiritual practice. Also, we are in a time and place where we are conditioned to have strong emotions and express them. Tantra encourages us to use those feelings and emotions as a meditative tool. When you touch into those strong emotions, you are very focused. Yuthok says that when your mind is sad, your meditation is very good. Usually, we want to distract ourselves from our emotions, but these teachings are designed to work with them. So we can laugh at ourselves for seeming a little shallow and perhaps initially turning toward tantra because we think it's about sex and massage and getting enlightened without much effort. But we can also celebrate ourselves for maybe instinctively knowing that this path is one that will help us during this time. In fact, maybe through being marketed as the fast track and being easily linked to enticing topics like sex, tantra knows exactly what it is doing to draw the busy and the lazy toward the practices that can heal us.

Whether sutra or tantra, there are antidotes to your poisons. There is a path for everyone. To begin, you could contemplate the Four Noble Truths for a few minutes each day as medicine for your mind. You could also contemplate the Buddha's story and how it symbolizes aspects of your own story. What palaces are you hiding within to avoid dealing with the realities of life? What stories of self arise when you are meditating? How does it feel to know that you possess the seed of Buddha Nature? How does it feel to know that every being possesses the seed of Buddha Nature? Considering all of this, what changes might you want to make to step onto the path? Further, you could apply the Four Noble Truths in your life as a regular remedy. You could notice times of suffering. You could notice the cause of that suffering—especially self-attachment. You could remember there is a cessation to suffering. You could apply the path—any of the practice tools that you will learn about in this book. Again, the Four Noble Truths is a basic medical model designed by an enlightened doctor, the Buddha, and it serves as a prescription for us all to heal our mental poisons and reveal the buddha within.

Just as you will often hear serious spiritual practitioners talk about their teachers with reverence and devotion, you will hear Buddhists talk about their lineages with respect and gratitude. In Buddhism, a lineage is a line of teachers, and their students, that practice a particular cycle of teachings over the course of generations. These lineages have a sustaining connection to the Buddha—the torch being passed from teacher to teacher. Sometimes, this torch is passed through visionary beings, even revealing teachings that have been hidden until it was the proper time for them to emerge, which only makes the continuation of the teachings all the more special. Buddhists often refer to fellow students in their lineage as their Sangha, or community. Because, to stay with the medical model, we don't just have the Buddha (and our teachers) as the doctor and the Dharma (the truth as disseminated through teachings and practices) as the medicine, we also have the Sangha as the nurse. This Sangha can mean all the noble enlightened beings preceding us who serve as an example. It can also mean all the noble students walking the path beside us right now.

It is not easy to course correct from wrong view to right view. We have a lot of conditioning supporting wrong view. However, we also have an extremely powerful doctor and medicine at our disposal along with our Sangha friends who can supply a spoonful of sugar to help the medicine go down. So, as you begin to take some of this medicine for the mind, please never feel that you need to do this alone. Talk with others about your efforts so you can laugh together about your obstacles. We all have a human mind. Again, there is nothing to be ashamed or afraid of here. Waking up can even be a good time. It turns out that right view—and the compassion and altruism it engenders—feels wonderful. Remember, we are moving toward health, happiness, and freedom.

"Remember your basic humanness."

- Dr. Nida Chenagtsang

Chapter Two – Yuthok's Two Treasures

Those interested in starting a serious spiritual practice often ask, "How do I find a teacher?" How do you find the doctor, medicine, and nurse of the Buddha, Dharma, and Sangha? When you have sincere aspiration, the teacher seems to find you. Practitioners often have serendipitous, even mystical, stories about connecting with a teacher, even in this day and age where anything under the sun can be found online. You can see in my own story that I somewhat magically stumbled into meeting with Sowa Rigpa medical studies and then the Yuthok Nyingthig spiritual path, only to find that it was what I had been looking for without even looking for it—this focus on nature, plants, health, and happiness. When we go searching for spiritual guidance and healing, we might not know what we are looking for or we might be looking for something very specific. If we make genuine wishing prayers and build up our spiritual bank account of merit, we might find ourselves finding a fit with a teacher and a path that feel like home, whether it all looks like what we imagined for ourselves or not. It's like love—it finds you.

Your wishing prayers and merit seem to be serving you well because, in this chapter, you will meet a genuine teacher. And it's not me. I am merely a messenger providing your introduction to Yuthok Yönten Gönpo. We will look at who Yuthok was, the overall path of the Yuthok Nyingthig, including brief descriptions of the main practices, and some basics of Sowa Rigpa in order for you to do an elemental typology self-assessment. However, there is no pressure to take Yuthok as your teacher. This is only a first date with Yuthok. Even better, Yuthok is not asking for monogamy. So, really, no pressure! The Yuthok Nyingthig practices may be what you want to explore as your main path, or they may become supplemental to other practices you do, or you may not want to practice them at all. This introduction might simply be a step to lead you to another teacher and path. Whatever happens, it is all good. Sometimes people hear about commitments you need to follow when practicing Tantric

Buddhism. And it is good to be committed to your spiritual practice. The only way for practice to work is to do it consistently and seriously. Moreover, there are some lineages that require certain commitments to a teacher or practice. But, with the Yuthok Nyingthig, you can relax your fears about these things. In fact, since its inception, it has been common for practitioners to explore the Yuthok Nyingthig as a supplemental path to boost their healing powers or as something to squeeze into their full lifestyle. You choose how you want to engage with Yuthok.

All of that said, it is important to comprehend the specialness of this moment. Meeting a teacher, even through a book, is a sacred event. These days, we have access to so many teachers and teachings that we can lose sight of the preciousness of receiving any teachings at all, especially as lay practitioners. When I started my spiritual path in earnest, I had a difficult time receiving teachings because I was not a monk. With my full schedule, I could not stay in a monastery for three months, so I could not get access to this or that teaching. I went through many hardships, like riding buses all day in the freezing cold only to be turned away at the door for being a layperson, but I tried my best to attain knowledge and then study and practice. When I think of my own story, I feel sadness for modern lay practitioners because we often do not receive important teachings. We might be told that we are not ready or we do not have the karma, and many times teachers are correct about this. To truly study and practice the teachings, we have to sacrifice time away from our normal lives and put in significant effort. But some of us may be prepared to do this even with our very full lives. I always thought that if I were to teach, I would do so in an easy and practical way to help as many people meet with this medicine as possible. I always think about impermanence—we never know when we will die. So I made a decision that while I am alive I want to share the medicine of Buddhism and Sowa Rigpa far and wide, making these teachings accessible to all humans. I like to inspire people to heal themselves and others from mental, energetic, and physical toxins. So now you are going to receive access to teachings that can help you do just that.

However, though you can relax your fears about commitments, I do want to emphasize one general commitment when approaching any spiritual path and especially Tantric Buddhism. Please remember that when you are a student, you are a student. I tend to be very encouraging with students because our world can be so disheartening and defeating. Also, many people suffer with the self's story of low self-esteem. So I want to empower students to trust themselves as practitioners and healers. However, I have found a negative aspect of motivating students, especially in cultures with strong conditioning in individualism, is they think they do not need a teacher. Students learn about Buddha Nature, or their inner guru, and maybe have interesting or pleasurable experiences while practicing, and then I hear them say, "I don't need a teacher. I'm my guru." This is unproductive and toxic thinking. It is spiritual materialism—poisonous pride dressing up in spiritual clothes. Ignorance runs very deep. Self-attachment is the strongest habit you have, so it will find all kinds of ways to avoid hearing the teachings and doing the practices. Self-attachment is like a toddler with its face scrunched up trying not to take the medicine. And that toddler, with a raging fever and snot-filled nose and hacking cough, is saying, "I'm my guru!" We all need a teacher to give us the teachings and help us with the practices. If you are a serious student, you receive teachings in a proper and respectful manner as befitting a serious education. None of us are realized buddhas—yet. If the disease is suffering and the path is medicine, you need a doctor to show you the way.

Of course, I am talking about working with real teachers—trustworthy, learned, generous, wise, humble, and compassionate teachers, not charlatans or abusers. One criterion for real teachers is they are real students. In a monastery, you might be a student for fifty or sixty years before you transmit teachings to the younger generation. In tantric lineages, it is the same. And, whether sutra or tantra, no matter how advanced your study and practice become, you always see yourself as a student and venerate your teacher, or guru, because they have essentially saved your life. Without your teacher, you would never receive the teachings. In some ways, your teacher is more important than even the Buddha because your teacher is here with you now, giving you the teachings. Therefore, because of this emphasis on the teacher-student relationship, it is important to take your time when choosing teachers and practices. You do not build a lasting, loving romantic relationship based on one date, right? Hello? No, you get to know someone. You see how your interactions make you feel and how the connection affects your life. It is the same with a spiritual teacher. The Buddha always encouraged students to explore the teachings and experiment with the practices rather than having blind faith in him or the path. Yuthok may be the right teacher for you, and I may be the right messenger for Yuthok—or not. If you are interested, then be a patient patient. Stay curious about the doctor and experiment with the medicine. Start slow and see how it goes.

YUTHOK YÖNTEN GÖNPO

Here is a big sign that Yuthok is not demanding monogamy from you—there are two Yuthoks. We have Yuthok the Elder and Yuthok the Younger. Yuthok the Younger is the teacher of the Yuthok Nyingthig and also considered to have compiled the four medical tantras, which collect the Sowa Rigpa teachings. He is the Yuthok we will discuss throughout this book.

However, it is important to also meet Yuthok the Elder, who is said to have been an ancestor of Yuthok the Younger. Yuthok the Elder was a semi-mythical figure of the eighth century. As such, we can talk about him in a practical or mystical way. For the practical among us, Yuthok's medical education began early, when he was selected for a children's program of sharp-minded students, without bias regarding background, to study Sowa Rigpa. Apparently, he was the best in the program and even bested older Tibetan doctors in tests of medical expertise. As an adult, he traveled to China, India, and the Middle East to gain information for Sowa Rigpa medical practices. This led to his being a prodigious author of medical texts and a renowned teacher and doctor. But it also played a role in his longevity as he is said to have traveled to all of these lands on foot. He did not want to torture animals, so he would not travel by horse or yak. He was a legend for not only his walking but also his strict diet. Among other austerities, he did not drink alcohol or eat meat, even supposedly saying that one needs to have a very stable meditation practice to do either. So he seems like a well-studied, sensible, and disciplined individual, known for his commitment to physical, emotional, and spiritual well-being. For the mystical among us, according to legends, his birth ushered in colorful rainbows and spontaneous music, and, as a child, he received visions of Medicine Buddha. In his middle age, after giving and receiving spiritual and medical teachings, he remained in meditation for three years and three months in a snow-covered mountain cave. He married at age 85 and had three sons who received his teachings. At age 120, he gave his final teaching and told his disciples he was going to Medicine Buddha's pure land where he would continue his healing activities, meaning he was going to physically die. Shortly thereafter, he and his wife and their dog (!) dissolved into light and rainbows—achieving the "rainbow body"—and the earth moved, rainbows appeared, and it rained flowers for three months. Achieving the rainbow body, with its accompanying natural displays, is a traditional sign of tremendous spiritual accomplishment. However you want to cut it, Yuthok the Elder was the real deal.

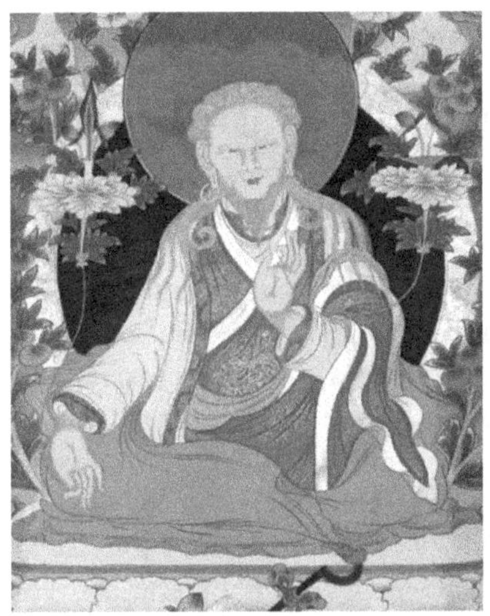

Yuthok Yönten Gönpo the Elder.

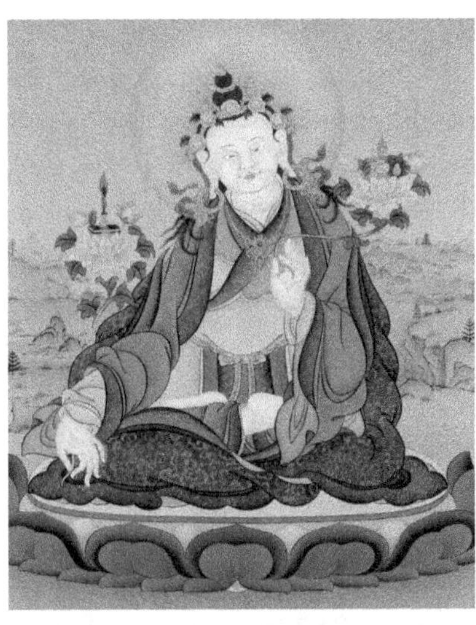

Yuthok Yönten Gönpo the Younger.

Yuthok the Younger also has the practical and mystical resume that is expected for precious teachers. He lived in the twelfth century and started his training in medicine and Buddhism during childhood, as he came from a long line of royal-court doctors. By fourteen, he was traveling through Tibet and receiving transmissions of medical tantras. As a young adult, he traveled to India to receive medical and spiritual teachings and is said to have returned six times. One of his noted teachers was the dakini—enlightened female being—Palden Trengwa who gave him the teachings and practices that would form the Yuthok Nyingthig. He established a medical clinic in Tibet and was an unparalleled physician, earning the name Yuthok Yönten Gönpo, which means the Lord of All Qualities. Like Yuthok the Elder, he was also an accomplished spiritual student and teacher, having visions of buddhas and demonstrating exceptional signs.

Once, while he was teaching at a governor's residence, fresh, golden arura fruits, the all-healing fruit of Medicine Buddha, fell within the walls of the residence for an hour. Of course, the audience rushed to get the fruits, even fighting among themselves. Yuthok let them know that had they not been so greedy, other special medicines would have rained down as well. Apparently, this kind of sign and others indicated that Yuthok's knowledge was unmatched, he had attained miraculous powers, and he was one with all the buddhas.

While that sort of story is special and magical and also ticks the traditional boxes of real-deal-ness, I am more drawn to Yuthok's humanity and approachability. As mentioned, he was known for his charity work— donating medicines to the sick and giving clothes to those in need. He was also known for being unfazed and nonjudgmental, essential qualities for a healer. Once, the king's daughter was very ill with gynecological issues, and no one could figure out why, especially because she would not talk about it. The truth was that she had masturbated with an old carrot and it had broken off inside of her. Yuthok suspected something of the sort and felt great compassion for the girl. He wanted to help her while also respecting her privacy. So he gave her some snuff that made her sneeze really hard, and the carrot shot out. Yuthok always said that if you had to choose between giving someone medical help or spiritual teachings, give them medical help because that could directly and immediately ease the suffering of a human life.

Fortunately, we do not have to choose between Yuthok's medical or spiritual offerings. Yuthok has left us two treasures—the Yuthok Nyingthig and the Gyü Zhi, the four medical tantras of Sowa Rigpa, which he is said to have compiled. The medical tantras discuss everyday physiology and psychology; they are geared for a general audience and medical professionals with the intention of delivering health and happiness in this life. The Yuthok Nyingthig is a spiritual text aimed at Tantric Buddhist practitioners pursuing complete liberation, or Buddhahood. It teaches meditation, ritual, and cultivation of the subtle anatomy, or energy body, as will be explained. This includes teaching the methods to accomplish the rainbow body. The rainbow body phenomenon and its associated practices thus have a strong connection with the Tibetan medical tradition.

How the Yuthok Nyingthig came to be composed is a beautiful story of the teacher-student relationship. Near the end of Yuthok's life, he traveled to Western Tibet, upon invitation by a local king, to deliver medical guidance and also a complete spiritual teaching of sutra and tantra. He brought his disciples and their family members, about 250 people, and the local residents and monks and nuns attended as well. For his teachings, Yuthok received many precious offerings, which he gave to the community, in addition to giving clothes, food, and medical treatments to those in need, as he always did—and always emphasized that his students do as well.

In that place, there was a temple with a statue of the Buddha. When Yuthok went to pay homage to the statue, a very powerful light radiated from the heart of the statue. Yuthok heard the mantra of compassion—OM MANI PADME HUNG—and also the mantra of Medicine Buddha—TADYATA OM BEKADZE BEKADZE MAHA BEKADZE RADZA SAMUDGATE SOHA. The light radiated out into the entire valley, which also filled with the smell of incense. Then the light came back and dissolved into the crown of Yuthok's head. At that moment, an earthquake shook the valley. It was a miracle. Everybody was shocked and in a state of commotion. Yuthok stayed silent in contemplation. Then he called his heart disciple, Sumtön Yeshé Zung, to him. Yuthok said he might soon depart for another land, meaning he would physically die. With the tremendous grief one feels over the physical loss of a teacher, Sumtön Yeshé Zung began to cry. Yuthok let him know it was too early for tears; he would live for some time, but he wanted to impart the lesson of impermanence. He encouraged Sumtön Yeshé Zung to not be lazy and instead ask questions and receive teachings now—never take your teacher's presence for granted.

Sumtön Yeshé Zung prostrated to Yuthok and praised him as the wish-fulfilling jewel that delivers the teachings, a unique and precious thing. Still rattled by the thought of losing his teacher, he asked Yuthok what his students should do without him when he eventually did depart.

Yuthok affirmed that receiving the teachings from a genuine teacher is the source of happiness in this world and also the key to becoming enlightened in a single lifetime—though, of course, this depends on the connection between student and teacher as well as the teacher's qualities and the student's courage, trust, and respect. But then Yuthok said there are many types of gurus, and it is important to understand them all. The first is your root guru who gives you an introduction to the true nature of your mind—Buddha Nature. The second guru is the lineage guru, meaning all of the teachers in your lineage. The third guru is the guru of texts, which is also known as the "black guru that never gets angry"—black from the ink smudging thanks to countless readings. The fourth guru is the guru of all phenomena—whatever exists in front of you, the five sensory experiences of sight, sound, smell, taste, and touch. In other words, your life. If you know life's true nature, everything is your guru. The fifth guru is the inner guru—your mind. In the end, your spiritual practice and health and happiness depend entirely on your mind. It is not suffering that is holding you; you are holding suffering. It is not your problems that are holding you; you are holding your problems. What is the nature of your pain and suffering? What is the nature of your problems? Look into this with your inner guru and liberate yourself from this grasping.

With renewed awareness of how precious it is to be with one's teacher, Sumtön Yeshé Zung continued his questions and ultimately asked for the teachings that would enable him to reveal Buddhahood in this lifetime. In response, Yuthok requested that Sumtön Yeshé Zung complete the uncommon Ngöndro, which you will learn about shortly. Sumtön Yeshé Zung practiced for several months and, out of appreciation, sold his land to make an offering of gold to Yuthok. When it was time for the teachings, Yuthok accepted the offering, which symbolized the wealth of the teachings, and gave the gold to those in need. Then he taught Sumtön Yeshé Zung the Guru Yoga practice and the entire path of the Yuthok Nyingthig. Sumtön Yeshé Zung transcribed the teachings in order to disseminate them to others. Yuthok then reviewed Sumtön Yeshé Zung's transcription of the teachings, and so the Yuthok Nyingthig was created for all beings, especially of this future time.

It is said that at age 76, Yuthok gathered his students for a final teaching before attaining the rainbow body and departing to Medicine

Buddha's pure land, the garden of Tanaduk, full of medicinal plants and herbs. There, he exists to support all of us for all time. And, because time and space are illusions, this means he is here with us right now. Yuthok, Medicine Buddha, and even Tanaduk are always on offer with all manner of healing powers whenever you choose to be aware of their blessings. Yuthok said that if you request his support and blessings, he will be there for you. Your teacher is always with you, displaying in everything you see and experience.

We use the word "vajra" a lot in Buddhism. A vajra is a ritual implement, and the word vajra is usually translated as indestructible. In fact, Tantric Buddhism is known as Vajrayana—the indestructible vehicle. This means that these teachings cannot be destroyed or defeated and they can take you all the way to liberation. I also like to translate vajra as indivisible. There is no original sin in Buddhism. Instead, there is the toxic ignorance of dualism, which is only a habitual confusion of mind; there is nothing original or permanent about it. So, if you are looking for something to blame for all suffering, then Satan is the mind's habit of subject-object separation and the Devil is the mind's habit of dualistic division. In fact, the word devil comes from the Greek word diabolos, meaning to divide or throw against. Thus, the only reason something could be destructible is if you mistakenly believe in its separate existence to be destroyed. Nothing is separate. Everything is connected. This is the teaching of emptiness. So your connection to your teacher is indestructible because it is indivisible. As you look for your teacher in everything, you see everything in everything. You rest in awareness of the indestructible indivisibility of it all. This awareness can bring with it experiences of great pleasure because you have given yourself a break from recreating the dualistic drama of self-other, or subject-object, which is the source of all your problems. A shorthand way of saying this in tantra is the subject is blissful and the object is empty—that is a pith instruction you can contemplate.

Eventually, this awareness becomes an experience of complete ease as even the oh-so-seductive sensation of pleasure further relaxes into states of loving kindness, compassion, joy, and equanimity. If you can comprehend that your teacher is always with you—not separate from you, but also not you—then your mind is flexible, and this path of awakening is working well for you. So Yuthok is here to be your teacher, your doctor, and everything you see, just as you are as well. That may sound a little strange, but don't worry. Out of his great compassion, Yuthok has developed a pragmatic and efficient set of practices for the busy and the lazy to deliver us into our natural and original state of bliss and Buddha Nature. So, with that, we will turn to an overview of the Yuthok Nyingthig.

YUTHOK NYINGTHIG

Here are the Yuthok Nyingthig practices displayed as a beautiful medicinal tree. I will now provide a brief introduction to the practices. Then the practices will be explored in the following three chapters as we look at which practices are best suited for which elemental types—wind, fire, and earth/water.

At the end of this chapter, you will be invited to complete an elemental typology self-assessment. Then you can explore the next three chapters—one dedicated to each type—knowing your elemental typology.

Regardless of your elemental typology, it would serve you well to read all of the chapters because: 1) any elemental type can have imbalances in any of the elements, 2) elemental imbalances can shift based on your location or lifestyle or stage in life, and 3) certain practices will only be discussed in certain chapters, and it is helpful to know about all of them.

Ngöndro

We already know that the preliminary practice of Ngöndro gives you a good childhood for your entire spiritual path. Accordingly, Ngöndro is displayed as the roots of the Yuthok Nyingthig tree. There are three Ngöndro practices. We already covered the common Ngöndro—the Four U-Turn Thoughts. Now, we will look at the uncommon Ngöndro and the routine Ngöndro.

The uncommon Ngöndro is uncommon because it is only for Buddhist practitioners. In many lineages, Ngöndro involves an enormous amount of accumulations—100,000 prostrations, 100,000 mandala offerings, and so on—that can take years if not an entire lifetime to complete. There is brilliance in this system as it builds devotion, reroutes

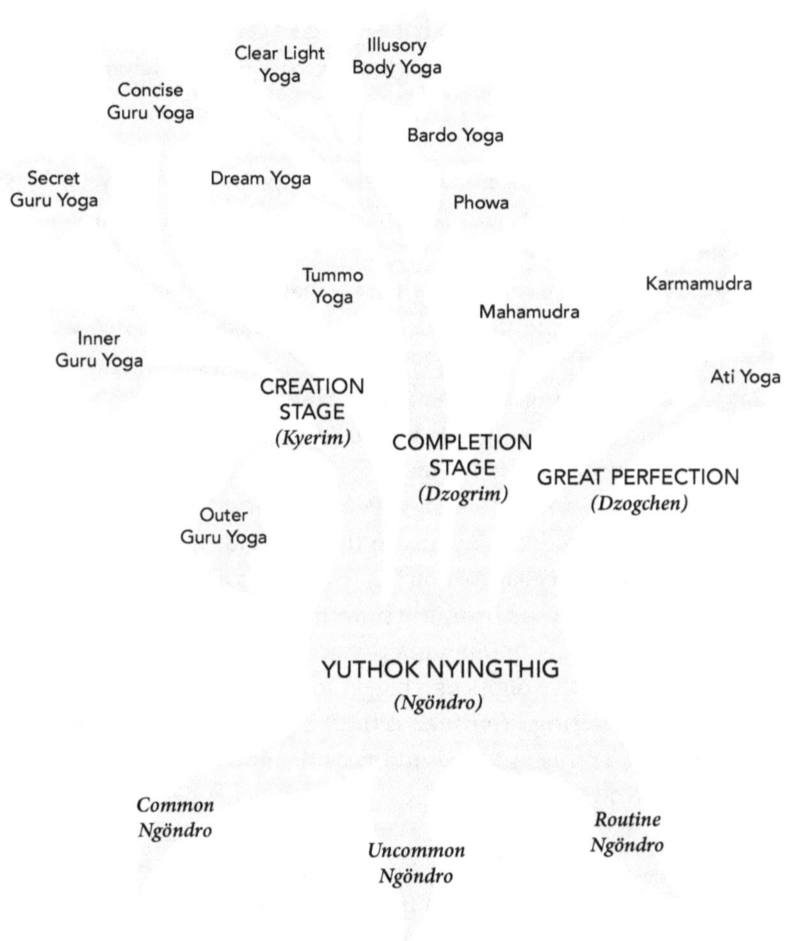

Clear Light
Yoga

Illusory
Body Yoga

Concise
Guru Yoga

Bardo Yoga

Secret
Guru Yoga

Dream Yoga

Phowa

Tummo
Yoga

Karmamudra

Mahamudra

Inner
Guru Yoga

Ati Yoga

**CREATION
STAGE**
(Kyerim)

**COMPLETION
STAGE**
(Dzogrim)

GREAT PERFECTION
(Dzogchen)

Outer
Guru Yoga

YUTHOK NYINGTHIG
(Ngöndro)

*Common
Ngöndro*

*Routine
Ngöndro*

*Uncommon
Ngöndro*

neural pathways, and crowds out samsaric activities that cause cyclical suffering. However, seeing as the Yuthok Nyingthig is designed for the busy and the lazy, our Ngöndro is designed to be a seven-day retreat. Do not be fooled by the shorter requirement. It is a potent practice and ideally repeated each year, like a battery recharge. The Yuthok Nyingthig Ngöndro involves several practices, and we will look at each one.

Refuge

The first practice is Refuge. People take refuge in many things. Maybe when you have problems with your partners, kids, friends, work, school, you smoke marijuana because it calms you down. You take refuge in marijuana. Or you get drunk, and then you have no worries, no memories, no problems. You take refuge in alcohol. People take refuge in love stories and get distracted from their problems by having fantasies, having sex, having arguments, things like that. People take refuge in work and money and success and get distracted from their problems by being on the phone, feeling important, and buying nice things. People take refuge in food, exercise, shopping, and technology. People even take refuge in anxiety, panic, and depression by returning to those mental states over and over. We do these things because we don't know what to do. We do these things again and again to escape from the suffering of human life, and then we create more suffering with our addictive and fruitless forms of refuge.

Refuge practice offers us a bigger form of refuge that can actually eliminate our suffering. You take refuge in the Buddha, Dharma, and Sangha. You take refuge in the Buddha as the doctor who is able to cure all problems. And you take refuge in Yuthok, your personal doctor on this path. You take refuge in the Dharma as the medicine that cures all problems. And you take refuge in your particular practice by doing it. You take refuge in the Sangha, which means the noble ones who are already enlightened and also your community of practitioners. Your spiritual friends are your nurses who often have to do the hard job, the dirty job, and give you the injections. Whether you see your friends as good people or bad people that is none of your business. Your focus is learning from your friendships and helping each other to do the practices. But, remember, the Buddha, Dharma, and Sangha can only show you the way; you have to walk the path yourself. So you take refuge here and now by saying it, meaning it, and doing it. You take refuge in the Buddha, Dharma, and Sangha until you get enlightened and can truly help others. There is a formal ceremony to take refuge, but a ceremony is only a ceremony. To really take refuge you examine the teachings and do the practices that work for you. That is best.

Bodhicitta

Bodhicitta is the mind that aspires to attain enlightenment for the benefit of all beings. Bodhisattvas are those who delay their complete liberation so they can keep returning to our world to be of benefit to all beings. Tibetan Buddhism, along with Buddhism in China, Japan, and the Himalayas, is part of the school of Mahayana Buddhism, which has an altruistic motivation at its heart. This means the practices train people to reveal bodhicitta and be bodhisattvas. So, at the start of all practices, you not only take refuge but also generate bodhicitta. You state that you do your practice for the benefit of all beings. Please take time to contemplate this. Usually in life, when we think we are being altruistic, we are still mostly concerned with ourselves. So please think deeply about how you are practicing this path to be of benefit to all beings.

You can further actualize this altruistic motivation by cultivating the Six Perfections of generosity, morality, effort, patience, meditation, and wisdom. The perfect meditation is calm abiding. The perfect wisdom is the insight into emptiness. With that perfectly calm and wise mind, you can skillfully display perfect generosity, morality, effort, and patience, which are the qualities required to do anything helpful and useful in this world.

So you generate bodhicitta by stating, and understanding, that you are practicing to be of benefit to all beings and then by doing your practices to cultivate the Six Perfections. Yuthok said that if you have an altruistic motivation, then whatever you do is Dharma practice.

The Four Immeasurables

With all the scientific knowledge in our world, there are still things you cannot measure—loving kindness, compassion, joy, and equanimity. These qualities are beyond science; they are limitless. In this practice, you cultivate unconditional love, universal compassion, infinite joy, and unending equanimity.

You meditate on your wish for all beings to have happiness and the causes of happiness—this is unconditional love. This is not our usual love that is like a business transaction. This is love without expectation or judgment or pushing or chasing.

You meditate on your wish for all beings to be free from suffering and the causes of suffering—this is universal compassion. Suffering can be mental, physical, old age, the suffering of suffering, changing suffering, all-pervasive suffering, and so on. People, animals, all beings are experiencing this cyclical suffering. You send your compassion to all beings, and it will help for sure.

You meditate on your wish for all beings to never be separated from the supreme joy that is beyond all suffering—this is infinite joy. You wish for all beings to feel the innate joy that we feel when we stop running around looking for joy outside of ourselves.

You meditate on your wish for all beings to abide in equanimity, free from attachment, aversion, and sorrow—this is unending equanimity. You wish for all beings to be completely content no matter what outer circumstances surround them. This is the equanimity within, which is a bottomless well of peace.

You say these wishes and meditate on them by bringing to mind specific people—people you love, people you hate, people you pass on the street. You can also make these wishes for people who have passed away. You can also make these wishes for animals and insects. You cultivate the Four Immeasurables for all beings across all time. You create a boundless state of bodhicitta.

For me, personally, the Four Immeasurables are the essence of this preliminary practice. If you have issues with any of the other practices, just focus on the Four Immeasurables.

Prostrations

Doing prostrations is a gratitude practice. The original prostrations were surya namaskar and chandra namaskar, sun salutations and moon salutations. You have probably heard of these or performed these in yoga class. Way back when, people would prostrate to the sun and the moon, thanking the sun for another day with light and the moon for another night with rest. These days, with the popularization of yoga, millions of people do sun and moon salutations, but they don't have gratitude for the sunlight and the moonlight. They do it so "I have a better back; I have a better ass; I feel good; I sleep good." I, I, I, I, I. There's nothing about gratitude for the sun and the moon. This is how ancient yoga traditions get corrupted; people make it all about themselves. It's okay—you can do that for exercise. But, if you really want to practice yoga, you need gratitude in your heart.

In Buddhism, we have guru namaskar. You prostrate to the guru, who, like a wish-fulfilling jewel, has given you the practices to liberate yourself. You feel so grateful for Yuthok because he gave us this wonderful, shortcut tantric practice. He thought about us in this future time and knew our problems. We are so busy with lives full of activities that give us trouble. We are so lazy with endless excuses about why we can't do spiritual practice. So, out of gratitude for Yuthok who created these amazing practices that can liberate the busy and the lazy, you do prostrations. You prostrate, say a prayer, and cultivate gratitude for Yuthok and the buddhas, gurus, teachers, parents, friends, everyone who helped you get to this place of good fortune to receive and complete these practices. You also visualize all sentient beings prostrating with you so they, too, receive blessings from your gratitude practice. You use your spiritual opportunity and power to send all beings loving kindness, compassion, joy, and equanimity through this practice of gratitude.

Mandala

Mandala offering is a generosity practice. You imagine everything you have and love—your body and possessions and joys and pleasures. You imagine everything everyone has and loves—their bodies and possessions and joys and pleasures. You imagine an entire universe of beauty and abundance. And you offer it all to the compassionate guru, Yuthok, over and over again. There is a prayer and a mudra (hand gesture) that you repeat as you offer and offer and offer. You offer everything from your heart. This is how you thank Yuthok for giving you these practices.

In return for your generosity, you receive wisdom and merit. Wisdom is the insight into interdependence and emptiness. Merit is spiritual energy. The Buddha said that before he did his six years of meditation, he needed to accumulate enough merit to make it possible. Merit can clear obstacles to practice and awakening. When you have wisdom and merit, you can do more practice and receive more results and benefit more beings. So the more you mentally offer to Yuthok, the more wisdom and merit you receive in return, and the more practice you are able to do, and the more benefit you are able to bring. We know this already from life—the more you give, the more you get. This is one way to stay balanced. Further, you can visualize all beings offering alongside you and receiving wisdom and merit in return. Again, you use your spiritual opportunity and power to send all beings loving kindness, compassion, joy, and equanimity through this practice of generosity.

Circumambulation

Circumambulation is a healing practice. You walk in a circle around a picture or statue of Medicine Buddha or anything representing Medicine Buddha, or you go for a walk and imagine Medicine Buddha on your right shoulder. While you walk, you say his mantra, audibly or silently— TADYATA OM BEKADZE BEKADZE MAHA BEKADZE RADZA SAMUDGATE SOHA. It is a mindful-walking exercise that is healing on multiple levels.

First, it is vital for humans to walk for at least thirty minutes every day. Both Yuthok the Elder and Yuthok the Younger were incredible walkers. They knew that daily walking promoted health and happiness. Often, when we dedicate a lot of time to spiritual practice, we are sitting; but we need to move as well. Because this lineage is focused on overall health, the uncommon Ngöndro uniquely includes circumambulation to make sure you get proper exercise while practicing.

Also, while circumambulating, you receive healing energy from Medicine Buddha as you connect with his presence and mantra. Through circumambulation, you develop a relationship with Medicine Buddha such that you can call on his support whenever you need help and healing. Moreover, you can visualize all sentient beings walking with you and receiving whatever healing they need from Medicine Buddha. Again, you use your spiritual opportunity and power to send all beings loving kindness, compassion, joy, and equanimity through this practice of healing.

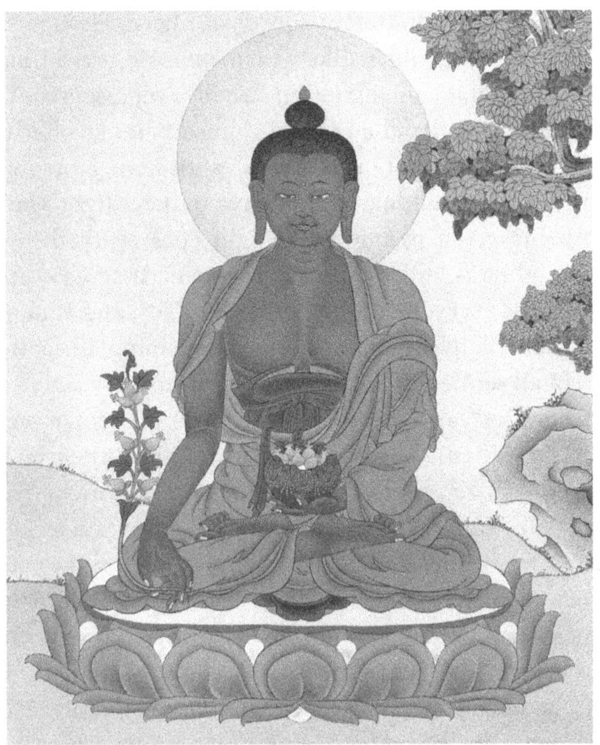

Medicine Buddha

Vajrasattva

Vajrasattva is also a healing practice. It is for healing, confessing, detoxing, and transforming. We cannot experience our Buddha Nature because our toxic emotions are so strong. It's like we are a crystal covered by cloudy confusion, muddy anger, grimy desire, stinky jealousy, and heavy pride. If you clean your mind of these emotional obscurations, there is more of a chance to experience your Buddha Nature.

To do this, you call upon Vajrasattva who is the yuthok purification deity in this body of tantric practices. Do you remember when you would get all worked up as a kid, upset about nightmares, fears, and worries? And a parent or loved one would place a hand gently on the top of your head. It soothed you and pacified you. That is Vajrasattva's energy.

So you visualize Vajrasattva above your head. He is made of white light, and he is wearing white silken garments. He is holding a vajra to represent indestructible compassion and a bell to represent the resounding clarity of emptiness. Light radiates from Vajrasattva as an offering to all the buddhas, and they offer light in return to Vajrasattva. Now supercharged with help from all the buddhas, Vajrasattva radiates light again, blessing all sentient beings. You imagine that light goes everywhere and heals everyone—all humans, animals, insects, spirits. It saves everyone from suffering. It brings everyone infinite happiness, joy, and equanimity. You are mentally, spiritually, and psychologically helping all sentient beings. Once you help all sentient beings, light returns to Vajrasattva and nectar pours from Vajrasattva's big toe and drips into the crown point of your head. The nectar of liquid or light washes through your entire body. Take your time to visualize and feel the nectar going to every inch of your body. It clears all emotional obscurations. Whatever you feel you need to confess, the nectar washes it out. Whatever negative energy you think you hold, the nectar washes it out. Whatever illness you think you have, the nectar washes it out. Whatever outside force you think is invading you, the nectar washes it out. Your sadness, anger, depression, jealousy, pride, attachment, the nectar washes it all out. Everything you wash out leaves through your eyes, nostrils, mouth, ears, pores, urethra, vagina, and anus. If you have garbage stuck in your head, now with Vajrasattva's nectar, please take it all out. If you want to do more meditation, then imagine in the earth there is a karmic-debt collector, a hungry spirit, who takes the garbage coming out of you as food. It all dissolves into nature and becomes compost, just like when we exhale carbon dioxide that is toxic for us but delicious for trees. Now you are filled with nectar, the nectar of joy. Your body is a stainless crystal, and your mind stays with joy. You say Vajrasattva's mantra while you do this. Please be egoistic during this practice; think of all your issues. Vajrasattva can clear them all out—for you and everyone.

Kusali Body Offering

Kusali body offering is another generosity practice. Don't worry, we only mentally offer our bodies. But still it can seem strange. So here are a few stories for context. First, the Buddha once offered his body. In one of the

Buddha's past lives, before he was the Buddha, he was a prince. One day, while hunting, he saw a tigress with many tiger-kitty babies. She was dying from starvation. He wanted to help her, so he cut his own flesh to feed her. She ate the flesh, was saved, and saved her babies. Second, Tibetans have a tradition of offering their dead bodies called sky burial. Here in the West, when somebody dies, you cremate or bury them. It is a way of saving part of our loved ones and even staying attached to them. In Tibet, after death, one of the most generous things you can do is offer your body to the animals. Your family brings your body to a specific place where professional people chop it up and feed it to the vultures. You know vultures only eat dead bodies. They are the trash collectors of nature, keeping everything clean and preventing disease. Sky burial is a final practice of generosity—a way to thank nature and animals for all that you have taken from them in your life. Finally, offering the body became a meditation tradition thanks to an eleventh-century female master, Machig Labdrön. She had been a super-intelligent little girl who was only interested in Dharma and trained in a monastery. As an adult, she had three children and lived as a single mother, which was very unusual and especially difficult at that time, and she still maintained her focus on Dharma. She created a practice called Chöd—to cut. In creating this practice, Machig Labdrön was coming from pure feminine wisdom, which is the realization of emptiness—interdependence and selflessness. Wisdom is considered feminine in Buddhism because it births the masculine of compassion. If you realize emptiness, you only act with compassion. So, in Chöd, from the wisdom of emptiness, you offer the main object of self-attachment in your life—your body—out of selfless compassion.

Our strongest attachment is to our bodies. Not our families, lovers, friends, houses, cars, careers, reputations—those are all secondary attachments. In the end, it will be your body that is very difficult to let go. The Buddha said that the body is the main troublemaker of self-attachment. We think about our bodies all the time. Mostly, we get angry with our bodies because they remind us of the reality of impermanence. Oh my skin, oh my hair, oh my wrinkles, oh my belly, oh I'm getting old, oh this and that. Even the pursuit of good health is self-attachment and body attachment. If you love yourself, that's good. You love yourself in a smart way. You treat yourself well. But let the body process life in its own way, too. Yes, you are getting older. Yes, you have more wrinkles. Yes, you have white hair. We don't want to get sick and age and have wrinkles and white hair because of attachment to the body. But the more you attach to your body, the more suffering comes—because everything that you don't want to happen will happen in life. You will age, get sick, and die. With wisdom, you can let your body go. Let your body disappear. Then you learn that after disappearance, there is appearance. There is appearing, disappearing, appearing; it is a circle. So, in Chöd, we feel the freedom of releasing attachment to the body by mentally offering it as a practice.

Here is how it works. You visualize your consciousness ejecting from your body and transforming into an enlightened, fiery-red female deity—a projection of your wisdom. Your body is imagined as a corpse that then becomes enormous, like a mountain. You, as the female deity, chop up your corpse, bless it with fire, wind, and water, and it becomes a vast ocean of nectar to offer. Then, out of compassion, you invite guests to the feast. First, you have the VIP guests of buddhas, and you offer this nectar to them with devotion. Next, you have Dharma protectors, a class of unseen beings who protect the teachings and practitioners; they are like the mob bosses of Dharma. You offer to them for protection for us all. Then, you offer nectar to the beings of the six realms of samsara—humans and animals and the unseen of gods, jealous gods, hungry ghosts, and hell beings. You offer to them out of compassion, giving them nectar that becomes whatever they desire—food, medicine, water, shelter, warmth, love. The needs of these beings are endless. You could give away billions of dollars and never even cover just human needs. With your infinite nectar, you can give and give and give—mentally, psychologically, and spiritually. There is no limit. Finally, you invite karmic debtor guests. These are wild and dangerous spirits, if you believe in spirits. These are demons and devils, if you believe in demons and devils. These are negative energies, if you believe in negative energies. These are people who frighten you, if you believe in fear. These are beings you owe in this life or past lives. Maybe in a past life you killed someone. Maybe in this life you built a house on top of a spirit's house. Maybe you cheated a friend out of some money. Maybe you did a lover wrong. These karmic debtor guests also include spirits connected with nature. And we have all cut their trees, contaminated their rivers, polluted their air. We have destroyed their forests, killed their wild animals, overfished their oceans. The more we take from nature, the more we are indebted to nature. These spirits do not have compassion; they are angry with us because we do stupid things. So, here, fearlessly you give back. You pacify them by offering blissful nectar to them. Even the vampire who wants to come and suck your blood—you say, "Please come, bring your family and your entire community to suck my blood." Rather than protecting yourself and fighting with others, there's no fight and no protection. From the wisdom of emptiness, you see the interdependence of how we all senselessly hurt each other, even others we can't see, in countless ways. So you drop your defenses. You break the cycle of suffering with the compassion of generosity. Here, take it; take it all. If you understand emptiness, there is no need to ever be scared of anything—people, animals, spirits, nature, neighbors, thoughts, feelings.

The question is whether our meditating and visualizing has an effect? For the mystical among us, wherever you send your mind, there is your energy. For the scientific among us, however you train your mind creates a neural pathway. For the pragmatic among us, whatever you are thinking informs your speech and actions, which impacts others, informing their thoughts and speech and actions. So you can create whatever kind of waves you want in your mind and in our world. Chöd helps you create internal and external waves of wisdom and compassion.

Ganapuja

At the end of the seven-day Ngöndro retreat, the busy and the lazy get to have a party. It's a spiritual party and also a confession practice. You gather with your sangha, offer food and drink to the buddhas and bodhisattvas and protectors, and mindfully enjoy the food and drink yourselves while you relax and talk. In this easygoing environment, you have the opportunity to resolve any issues with your sangha friends and teachers and even the buddhas, bodhisattvas, and protectors. You are all together, enjoying the same substances, seeing the best in one another, and letting things go.

Routine Ngöndro

Routine Ngöndro is a lifelong practice of promoting positive waves in our world. It follows the Buddha's instructions to strive for good deeds as much as possible, avoid negative actions as much as possible, and tame your mind. Routine Ngöndro is unique to the Yuthok Nyingthig, which has a strong emphasis on bringing practice into the world through medicine and healing of all kinds—not just sitting on a meditation cushion. When engaging in routine Ngöndro, it is important to infuse compassion with wisdom so you hold a long-term, interconnected view to promote what is truly beneficial as opposed to what might be enabling unproductive or unhealthy habitual actions. There are six aims:

1. Be involved in charity projects that help individuals who are experiencing a lack of resources and/or illness.

2. Find ways to save the lives of people and animals.

3. Always strive to spread the Buddha's and Yuthok's teachings, especially the medical tantras and the Yuthok Nyingthig.

4. Create a clinic or center where those who are in need can receive help.

5. Make donations or offer your time to help build things that will benefit many beings such as community centers, animal shelters, or infrastructure projects supporting health and safety.

6. Take care of abandoned animals and protect the environment.

Empowerment

Traditionally, after Ngöndro, you receive an empowerment to then begin creation stage and completion stage practices. An empowerment is a ritual where the teacher empowers you to practice a certain practice or set of practices, which could involve regenerating as a buddha or deity. As such, pursuing a practice is the only reason to receive an empowerment. There is no need to collect empowerments; they are not for spiritual shopping and entertainment. In the Yuthok Nyingthig, we have a two-day empowerment and an essentialized empowerment, which is much shorter. We are going to discuss creation stage and completion stage practices in this book; however, please know, that in order to truly understand and practice creation stage and completion stage you need to receive an empowerment from a qualified teacher.

In your aspiration to receive an empowerment, the proper motivation is bodhicitta, as always. You aim to deepen your practice and cultivate the Four Immeasurables so that you can free all beings from suffering. The proper container for this bodhicitta is gratitude. To find Tantric Buddhism and have access to these teachings is like someone who is experiencing poverty digging through a trash heap and stumbling upon a wish-fulfilling jewel. In fact, we have been digging through the garbage of samsara looking for satisfaction in all the wrong places—outside of ourselves in our never-ending human desires. But now, you have the precious opportunity to uncover the real thing—the great bliss of Buddha Nature that will liberate you from endless wanting and completely cease your suffering. In so doing, it will transform you into the buddha you truly are, capable of helping any being at any time in exactly the manner they need to liberate as well. You have wandered for so long; I know because I have, too. I feel so fortunate to have received this Tantric Buddhist education. This path is so beautiful. We learn many things in life; we are very educated. Many of these things you learn with your head. But with tantra, you learn with your head and heart in a unified way. When I was young, I would read these texts and I would cry. And normally I am not a crying guy. But when I study and practice tantra, I have tears of joy because I am so lucky. I feel so fortunate to have the karma to receive these teachings and do these practices. I received teachings from so many schools and then found that the Yuthok Nyingthig had put them all together. It is truly an amazing path; you can feel it with your heart. So I offer my small story as an example of how you could approach any empowerment with gratitude.

Once you are feeling lucky, happy, and ready to make this tantric journey, the empowerment helps you to become more open. Before empowerment, you are unripe—solid and hard and fixed. Because of empowerment, you ripen and soften and start to recognize your true nature; your wisdom matures. This gift of growth comes from the teacher who provides a guided meditation to open your chakras, or energy centers. You visualize the meditational deity of the empowerment, in this case the guru Yuthok, and receive light from the deity's chakras to your chakras— head, throat, heart, navel, base. Receiving this light blessing clears each chakra's toxins, revealing their innate elemental balance. Your ignorance, attachment, anger, pride, and jealousy become space's spaciousness, fire's awareness, water's clarity, earth's equanimity, and wind's activity that puts them all to perfect use. Your mind, speech-energy, and body transform; you become rainbow-like. During empowerment, it is possible to enter into a state of bliss. This is your original state where you can experience Buddha Nature.

When you are in this original and blissful state, you are free from all mental toxins. Maintaining this state is tantra, which also means continuation. From the blessing of your teacher and their teachers and their teachers, you receive a living transmission that calls forth your inherent Buddha Nature—and this is the uninterrupted lineage blessing of tantra. It is a wave, moving through all of us and everything. Like a river, let it flow. Like the wind, let it blow. Like the snow, let it fall. Like a bird, let it fly. Like a flower, let it blossom. Like life, let it happen. Let it all happen, mindfully, joyfully, blissfully. When your mind is focused on bliss and joy, there is only bliss and joy.

When the Buddha became enlightened, he was attacked by the maras, but their weapons became flowers. The Buddha didn't use a shield. He didn't escape. He just sat there. Once we master the mind, we master the elements and the external world. Empowerment invites us into this mastery. It gives us permission to follow in the footsteps of the Buddha and all the great masters. Then we can be of benefit to all beings—because, in our Buddha Nature, we see and treat all beings as the buddhas they truly are.

Creation Stage and Guru Yoga

Guru Yoga is a regular practice of self-empowerment that is vital to Tantric Buddhism. Essentially, you visualize the meditational guru of your practice, meditate on your teacher's oneness with the guru, and receive light blessings from your guru/teacher to your five chakras, similar to the empowerment ceremony. It is very powerful medicine that clears your toxins and balances your energy. It can feel like taking an energetic shower, as you might be awash in bliss. Yuthok said Guru Yoga is the great enhancer and accelerator—the guru's blessing speeds up the fruition of all the other practices you do.

One reason this practice accelerates other practices is because Guru Yoga cultivates gratitude. It is an opportunity to feel deep appreciation for your teachers and their teachers and all the teachers who have helped you receive the teachings and do the practices. On your own, none of this learning and awakening would be possible. Out of loving kindness and compassion, your teachers have done the work to be of benefit to all beings, and you are now reaping the rewards of their efforts. If you can find this gratitude in your Guru Yoga, then it will allow for faster results in all of your practices.

Further, through Guru Yoga, you deepen your connection with the continuation of tantra, the awakening of blissful Buddha Nature within all beings throughout time and space. Whenever you do this practice, it is a precious opportunity to add to the overall awakened energy in our world. With this understanding, you maintain bodhicitta throughout Guru Yoga and cultivate wishes for loving kindness, compassion, joy, and equanimity for all beings. Of course, you can imagine all beings doing Guru Yoga with you. This altruism within Guru Yoga also amplifies the efficacy of all of your practices.

Finally, the Guru Yoga of the Yuthok Nyingthig is an especially great accelerator because Yuthok asked for it to be so. He explained this to Sumtön Yeshé Zung before he transmitted the Yuthok Nyingthig. Yuthok said that the kindness of all buddhas is the same; they all have the same blessing energy. But they each had their own aspirations when they became a buddha. Medicine Buddha was a human, an ordinary being. When he awakened to Buddhahood, he asked to eliminate disease for all sentient beings. That was his last wish and that is why he became Medicine Buddha. Avalokiteshvara, the buddha of compassion, wished to transmit love and compassion to all sentient beings. Manjushri, the buddha of wisdom, wished to help all sentient beings wake up through their wisdom. Vajrapani, the buddha of power, wished to bestow positive power upon all sentient beings because we need serious strength to liberate ourselves. Tara, a female buddha, wished to eliminate obstacles for all sentient beings. Yuthok's last wish was fast blessing. He wanted to accelerate the fruition of practices because he knew humans would become increasingly busy and lazy—busy with samsaric problems and lazy for spiritual practice. He knew that we would have less courage and stamina for spiritual practice. So he wanted to give the gift of essentialized practices that could bring results quickly for students. Yuthok said that if somebody does one week of this practice with sincerity and without distractions, they will see him in person or in visions or in dreams and he will give them directly whatever practice and instructions they need. On that note, Yuthok also emphasized that you don't need to practice with many buddhas because all buddhas are in one buddha. Any buddha you choose for any practice will include all the powers and blessings of all the buddhas. Buddhas only appear to have different blessings to connect with different types of people. Remember, there are 84,000 antidotes to our 84,000 toxins. In fact, you can do the Yuthok Nyingthig Guru Yoga while visualizing a meditational guru other than Yuthok—provided it is a guru within this tradition of Tantric Buddhism and thus available for Guru Yoga. While Yuthok is not a monogamist, consent is always necessary. So if you have another guru within the Tantric Buddhist tradition, that is wonderful—stay with what is easy and appealing for you.

The Yuthok Nyingthig Guru Yoga is also particularly important and speedy because it combines creation stage practice with Guru Yoga. Last chapter, we discussed creation stage practice—you regenerate as a buddha to remind yourself of your Buddha Nature, to even experience your Buddha Nature, and to course correct from your ignorance at rebirth when you habitually generated the dense form of a human despite actually being a buddha, like every other being. So, during Guru Yoga, you regenerate as a buddha and then receive the light blessing from Yuthok, or whatever guru supports your path. And that personal choice extends to your own regeneration. Of course, there are buddhas suggested for the creation stage aspect of Yuthok's Guru Yoga—usually to recreate yourself as Medicine Buddha or a union of buddhas. But you can recreate yourself as any buddha or deity you would like if you are already working with one from another lineage and/or practice within Tantric Buddhism. In giving us this freedom during practice, Yuthok helps us stop shopping for buddhas. In our laziness, we can become busy chasing after this and that, including chasing after buddhas and deities and practices. Yuthok knew that humans could get lost in the chase and never actually do any practice. So Yuthok said stick with one—one for your creation and one to transmit the light blessing. Whatever works for you, stick with it. Just please do the practice.

The Yuthok Nyingthig has four Guru Yogas. The Outer, Inner, and Secret Guru Yogas are each practiced as a seven-day retreat, but each one can also be a daily practice. The Concise Guru Yoga is mainly a daily practice. Outer Guru Yoga connects you with the outer guru, Yuthok, building your relationship with the lineage and increasing your openness to receive blessings. Inner Guru Yoga connects you with your inner guru, showing you the buddha you truly are. Secret Guru Yoga connects you with your innate bliss and wholeness, your unconditioned original state. Concise Guru Yoga includes all of this and also a long-life practice.

A final reason why Guru Yoga is essential to the Yuthok Nyingthig is because it serves as a form of Shamatha, or calm abiding, meditation. Creation stage practice is the calm abiding meditation of the tantric path. Humans have 65,000 thoughts per day; cool-looking people have more. And these thoughts are the basis of your mental suffering. Regardless of what is actually happening to you, it is the thoughts about it all that drive you out of your mind. Actually, your thoughts drive you too deeply into your mind, yourself, and your blah blah blah. You try to escape your thoughts, but you cannot escape them. You cannot escape your own mind. And most of our thoughts are automatic—like unstoppable waves upon waves. So, to heal our mental suffering, we need to deal with our thoughts. Shamatha meditation is best for this; it is the overall immune-boosting practice. It calms the waves of thoughts; it eases your mental symptoms. Then you can see what specific toxins need to be healed. Is it desire? Is it anger? Is it confusion? Is it jealousy? Is it pride? That way, you can get to the root of the infection with the powerful antivirals of completion stage. Remember or imagine that calming, loving adult hand on top of your head when you were a child, all worked up and scrunched up and not wanting to take the medicine. The blessing of the guru settles you down, giving the medicine a fighting chance to heal you once and for all.

Completion Stage

With creation stage, you recreate yourself into the buddha you actually are. You recreate your body, your speech-energy, and your mind. With completion stage, you realize that everything is complete within yourself. Everything is perfect internally. You do not need to look outside of yourself for anything—including enlightenment. You can wake up as you are. In the Yuthok Nyingthig, there are six yogas within completion stage. We have two yogas for the daytime, two yogas for the nighttime, and two yogas for death. These practices will be briefly explained here, and some will be covered more in the following chapters depending on whether they are especially beneficial medicine for balancing wind, fire, or earth/water.

The daytime yoga practices are Tummo Yoga and Illusory Body Yoga. Tummo Yoga shows you that the ultimate nature of human sensation is blissful heat. It is a physical practice ideally done at dawn. In the morning, when the sun is rising, your tummo heat naturally rises as well. You feel joyful and happy. If you are not arising in the morning feeling naturally joyful and happy, it is a sign that your inner pilot light is diminished; thus, it is very important to find and do spiritual practices that work for you—stat! Tummo Yoga helps you notice, experience, and cultivate the self-arising blissful heat of the body. This bliss is the true nature of your inner energy. This bliss is what you could experience all day. With your tummo fire warming your being, you enter into your day with happiness. Then you practice Illusory Body Yoga throughout the day. This is a fantastic practice for releasing self-image and body-image issues. Illusory Body Yoga helps you understand the illusion of the self by understanding the illusion of the body. You come to see all the ways you create a self—the self of here and now, the self in your thoughts, the self in your memories, the self in your fantasies, the self in your dreams, the self on social media, the self in others' thoughts about you. All of these selves have bodies that you imagine, including the self and body of the here and now. Through this practice, you can learn that you are actually made of light that is constantly shape shifting, as is everything. This illuminates the utter illusory ridiculousness of your thoughts about you, others' thoughts about you, and your thoughts about others' thoughts about you. So, through these two daytime yogas, you come to know your energy is bliss, your body is light, and your self-image and body image are mental habits that cause a lot of pain for you and everyone around you and our world. Please, don't make life heavy—make it light.

Then, at night, you go to sleep. Once you fall asleep, there are two yogas for the nighttime. While you are dreaming, you can do Dream Yoga. Your dreams are a good barometer for your mental and emotional health; they show you what is going on down in your depths, which is often hidden to you during the day. Through Dream Yoga, you can free yourself from the subtlest activity of mind and energy by becoming lucid in your dreams. This means that you catch and transform your dreams; you make your dreams into whatever you would like. Mastering your dreams in this manner frees you from toxic thoughts and emotions, even those buried deep down; this, in turn, helps you master your life. Further, dreaming is a middle state between deep sleep and waking, similar to the bardo—the middle state between death and rebirth. Dream Yoga is good practice for maintaining awareness in the bardo so you do not habitually run right into the next hamster wheel of suffering. Clear Light Yoga is for the deep sleep state of no dreams. During deep sleep, your sense of self completely dissolves; you are in ultimate freedom. This is good practice for death when it is possible to achieve total liberation by realizing your innate light. If you miss this opportunity at death, then you enter into the bardo. During Clear Light Yoga, you maintain awareness of dissolving into the clear light every night so you are ready to do this with ease upon death.

When we are done repeating day and night, we reach our final day. It's called death. And it can come in the day or the night. For death, you also have two yogas. For the moment of death, you have Phowa, which is the process of ejecting the consciousness consciously. You can practice this process during life. It will help you die in peace and travel to a pure land—a state of being where it is effortless to reveal enlightenment. Then you can practice Bardo Yoga, which enables you to make a conscious choice for your rebirth into a form and a life that will be beneficial for all beings. This, too, can be practiced during life and familiarizes you with the process of dying such that you have freedom and choice after death.

Karmamudra, Mahamudra, and Ati Yoga

The final branches of the Yuthok Nyingthig tree contain three practices. Karmamudra and Mahamudra are on one branch of completion stage, and Ati Yoga is the branch of the Great Perfection (Dzogchen in Tibetan). Tibetan Buddhism has four different schools with slightly different methods. The Yuthok Nyingthig, being nonsectarian, includes methods from a couple of the schools. Karmamudra and Mahamudra come from one school and Ati Yoga from another. But they are all doorways into the same room. There are 84,000 medicines.

These practices will be discussed in the coming chapters. For now, it is important to comment on the popular appeal of these practices. In general, people like to rush into so-called higher-level practices, especially in tantra, because these practices are enticing in their seeming simplicity and even sexiness. Gone are the complex visualizations and complicated methods. The deeper you go in tantra, the easier the practices become in terms of form. Maybe you already know this, and this is why you have come to tantra—to take it easy. Maybe you have heard Mahamudra and Ati Yoga are all about doing nothing. Maybe you have heard Karmamudra is all about getting off. But if you say, "Oh good, I can relax and have orgasms and get enlightened. I don't need the complicated practices. I can just do these easy ones," then you are not yet ready for these practices. First of all, you are missing the point. Second, when your mind is flexible, you are okay with complexity and you are okay with simplicity. You are okay with everything. You are not selective. When you are selective, that is a problem. You are still choosing. You always want something good for yourself, easy for yourself. You are still searching and running around.

Moreover, some people receive high teachings and think they can just do these practices; they no longer need to spend time and effort on Guru Yoga. But the heart of these practices is devotion and bodhicitta—exactly what we cultivate in Guru Yoga. It is your connection with your teacher and your compassion for all beings that unlock the doors of these so-called higher-level practices.

So let's talk about devotion. Devotion is all about gratitude. You are grateful that the Buddha discovered and shared these teachings. You are grateful that Yuthok simplified them for this time. You are grateful to have made a connection with these practices. You are grateful to have the time and leisure to do these practices. You are grateful for all of the humans and events and circumstances that have gifted you this opportunity. You want to do something of true value with your life. You want to wake up so you can do something of actual benefit for our world, not something motivated by pride or greed or reputation but motivated by loving kindness and compassion.

With this devotion, you will begin to reveal bodhicitta. At first, you will reveal bodhicitta on the relative level. As you practice, you will start to feel good. You will bathe in happy hormones, inviting unprecedented ease and relaxation. While practicing, your problems and sufferings will slip away because you cannot experience blissful pleasure and samsaric pain at the same time. Moreover, you will know that this joyful state depends on nothing other than being. You will see the deep confusion of humans as we chase this and that, causing endless problems for ourselves and others. You will break open with a love for all beings that you have not known before, and your awakened heart will radiate. You will create a field of spacious awareness, stillness, peace, and joy. You will move toward revealing ultimate bodhicitta and existing in a state of compassionate creativity and altruistic responsiveness at all times. You will move toward realizing freedom for us all.

Human beings are actually very kind animals. Watch children. They have such tender emotions and want to care for each other. When we are small and still relatively unconditioned, we want to be happy, have friends, and play. When we see animals or people suffering, we have innate love and compassion for them. We want to save a little animal, save a little bug, save a little flower—these are little gestures of our love and compassion. Remember your basic humanness. So many of us lose touch with this quality and then try to build up superficial power, even superficial spiritual power. It is a sad wrong turn, motivated by confused wrong view. This is why we focus so much on bodhicitta from the start of this path. Bodhicitta is the root and the trunk and the fruit. Any practice you do, start with the Four Immeasurables—loving kindness, compassion, joy, and equanimity. Then you will become calm and humble. Then you will be of benefit.

Everything you are looking for is within you. Tantric Buddhism is as vast as an ocean; it is easy to get lost. Thankfully, Yuthok has given us this simple path back home.

SOWA RIGPA

Because we are traveling this path in our human bodies, Yuthok, out of his great compassion, has given us his other treasure—Sowa Rigpa, the science of health and happiness. In this section, we will look at the basic aims of Sowa Rigpa and the role of the elements in your well-being. At the end of this section, you will be invited to complete an elemental typology self-assessment, which will inform your exploration of the rest of this book as we discuss diet and lifestyle modifications as well as spiritual practices best suited for each elemental type.

As stated, Sowa Rigpa has a fourfold aim—preventing illness, curing illness, extending life, and cultivating happiness. When you are healthy, you need to know how to maintain good health. When you are not healthy, you need to seek support. These days, many people have an aversion to medicine and doctors. But medical science should be a part of our lives because medical science is all about enjoying life. Each and every one of us needs to know about medical science because ultimately you are your own doctor, just as ultimately you are your own spiritual teacher. In fact, tantra, or body protection, was originally a medical term. Later, it became used for spiritual purposes. In the West, tantra has become sexy. In Tibet, tantra is boring. It's about taking care of a human body. And this is something we have to do each and every day—remember, tantra also means continuation. You need to know how to care for your mind and body in order to make life easier and more enjoyable for you and everyone around you.

Sowa Rigpa makes medical science user-friendly and fun. When people hear about Sowa Rigpa in the West, it can seem like a whole new big thing to learn. But Sowa Rigpa is really about reminding ourselves of our natural human instincts. If we listen to our bodies, we are already practicing Sowa Rigpa. That said, without clear instructions and explanations, we often get confused and don't trust ourselves. Again, as with spiritual practice, though you are your own teacher, you always need a teacher. So learning about Sowa Rigpa is a process, but it's more like relearning or remembering or revealing. In fact, revealing your inner health and happiness is not unlike revealing your inner bliss and freedom. It's all inside, waiting to shine. You can live long and have fun and be free.

According to Sowa Rigpa, humans are supposed to live for about 100 years. We die early because of disease, accidents, and suicide. These days, the leading causes of early death are mainly lifestyle diseases that can be prevented. Indeed, chronic disease is often due to our losing patience with prevention. Barring accidents beyond our control, living for 100 happy-and-healthy years comes down to taking care of ourselves.

Yuthok the Elder said we are all born with ten good batteries, each capable of giving us ten good years. As it is with your mobile phone or computer, if you misuse your batteries, you will die sooner. So you need to learn how to preserve your personal battery power. For example, physical activity can preserve battery power. Most of us are too sedentary and could use more exercise to boost our batteries. However, some of us overdo it with physical activity. Our extreme exercising can overuse our batteries and shorten our lives. Sowa Rigpa helps you understand your personal needs so you can find the right balance with food, herbs, sleep, rest, movement, exercise, sex, work, relationships, community, nature, and spiritual practice—all the things that affect our batteries.

In Sowa Rigpa, at the heart of our personal needs, is a need to care for the mind. Sowa Rigpa holds the same view as the original doctor on this path, the Buddha, that the primary cause of illness is the three mental toxins—desire, anger, and ignorance. Because of desire, anger, and ignorance, we do things that lead to the secondary causes of illness— unsuitable diet, unsuitable lifestyle, not being in harmony with time/ seasons, and not being in harmony with nature, other humans, and even spirits. In other words, when we are suffering with mental toxins, we have thoughts, say things, and take actions that cause further suffering, including illness, for ourselves and then others. Recall the U-turn thought of cause and effect. Today's energy, mood, and health depend on yesterday's thoughts, speech, and actions.

For example, let's say you are consumed by desire. You want things—a partner, a different partner, sex, stuff, money, attention, and so on. And, not getting these things, you try to fill this sense of need with sugary food. This leads to physical problems of poor digestion, weight fluctuation, bone deterioration, tooth decay, liver toxicity, skin and hair dryness as well as mental problems of mood swings, anxiety, lack of focus, and so on. Or, let's say you are consumed by anger. You are raging—against your parents, your partner, your former partner, your boss, your clients, the person next to you in traffic, and so on. And, unable to calm down, you exercise every free moment you have. This leads to physical problems of poor digestion, joint wear-and-tear, aging skin, hair loss, menstrual issues, and fatigue as well as mental problems of distraction, stress, competition, aggression, and so on. Or, let's say you are consumed by ignorance. You are avoidant—of people, work, change, emotions, and so on. And, unable to look at life, you are hiding in food, media, information, and sleep. This leads to physical problems of poor digestion, weight gain, swollen joints, low libido, and lethargy as well as mental problems of sadness, depression, loneliness, and so on. In the Introduction, we played out these toxic cause-and-effect scenarios more fully. You get the picture. You can U-turn your health by working with the three mental toxins of desire, anger, and ignorance, which we all have in different proportions.

Enter the elements. Because here's the big secret—you get to blame something for your mental toxins. Humans love to blame things other than ourselves. And Buddhism is such a drag because it's all about taking responsibility for your mind and life. But now here's your chance! You can blame the arising of desire, anger, and ignorance on your elemental imbalance. Oh, I'm not needy; it's wind imbalance. Oh, I'm not aggressive; it's fire imbalance. Oh, I'm not in denial; it's earth/water imbalance. In all honesty, this is real. According to Sowa Rigpa, elemental imbalances lead to energetic, mental, and physical issues—and, again, the primary issue is mental toxins compelling us into all kinds of suffering. Jokes aside, blaming the elements can also help us have compassion for ourselves and others. It puts a little space between ourselves and our issues, not to mention a little space between ourselves and others' issues. If we want to be Buddhist about it, we can contemplate the emptiness of self—there is no static and solid "I" at all, just an interplay of elements that can lead to displays of thought, speech, and action that are of pain or pleasure, contraction or expansion, conditioning or freedom, harm or benefit, all depending on imbalance or balance.

In fact, it is emptiness that explains how the elements are affecting us. Sowa Rigpa holds the same philosophical view of Buddhism that nothing can exist by itself, entirely separate or independent from the rest of the universe. All phenomena are connected to one another through interdependent cause-and-effect, linked together in a vast web. And everything in that web is comprised of the building blocks of the five elements—space, wind, fire, earth, and water. The five elements are the materials from which all life in all universes originates. These elements are present in our bodies as well as our environments, our planet, our galaxy, and on and on. Everything you see is some combination of these elements. The three elemental energies of our bodies—wind, fire, and earth/water—are born from the interplay of these elements with the fifth element of space. And these elemental energies are also the bridge between mind and body, the basic force that makes mind and body work, or not work.

So, in Sowa Rigpa, we use elemental typology to look at your nature and how to balance it. This method of exploring health and healing through typologies is not unique to Sowa Rigpa. The Greek system has four humors. The Ayurvedic system has three doshas. Sowa Rigpa has three elemental energies. This is all part of a universal, natural medicine tradition. We need never argue about which specific branch of the tradition is better. All types of medicine can help. When healing self and other, we need to use whatever the patient needs. And, in Sowa Rigpa, your typology can tell you what your body needs and what your mind needs—and how to meet these needs with compassion. Elemental typologies are beautiful, not to mention vital. When you face mental and physical challenges, you don't need to blame the elements; you just need to balance them.

To that end, here's how the primary cause of illness—the three mental toxins—breaks down by elemental imbalance. Desire and attachment is the result of a wind imbalance. Anger and aggression is the result of a fire imbalance. Ignorance and confusion is the result of an earth/water imbalance. When we don't know how to balance the element into vital nectar, we poison self and other. However, you can build lasting health and happiness by knowing your nature and making slow and steady changes to balance your elements. Generally speaking, wind imbalance needs to care for the nervous system; fire imbalance needs to decrease inflammation; earth/water imbalance needs to address metabolic issues. Another way to say this is: wind types need nourishing; fire types need detoxing; and earth/water types need fasting. This means nourishing, detoxing, and fasting holistically across mind, speech-energy, and body. Then we can transform the poisons of desire, anger, and ignorance into vital nectars of awareness, clarity, and spaciousness. We can see and feel that everything is really okay, even good, even blissful. We can have the ultimate flowers and fruits of Sowa Rigpa—the two flowers of good

BODILY CHARACTERISTICS

CHARACTERISTICS	WIND	FIRE	EARTH / WATER
Height	Shorter	Average height	Taller
Weight	Underweight; easily loses and struggles to gain weight	Average weight; easily maintains weight	Overweight; struggles to lose and easily gains weight
Physical Build	Small, slender, skinny, delicate	Medium build, muscular	Stout, heavy-set, big bodied, big limbs
Posture	Stooped, hunched spine	Erect spine and posture	Open-chested, arched spine, swayed back posture
Joints	Protruding; crack easily when moving	Average; well-formed	Less prominent; well-hidden under skin, muscle, and fat
Skin and Complexion	Darker or bluish complexion; dry, rough, flaky skin	Yellowish or reddish complexion; oily skin prone to inflammation and breakouts	Pale or light complexion; soft, smooth, plump, well-hydrated skin
Hair	Dry, thin, rough	Oily; blond or reddish in color	Thick, luxurious, voluminous; well-hydrated; thick eyelashes
Body Temperature	Irregular; sensitive to cold, windy weather and temperature fluctuations	Runs hot; sweats easily and a lot	Generally, consistently cold but insensitive to temperature changes
Digestion, Metabolism	Inconsistent, sensitive digestion	Strong digestion and metabolism	Slow metabolism and sluggish digestion
Appetite	Irregular	Strong, consistent thirst and appetite	May not feel strong appetite but snacks habitually
Favorite Tastes and Foods	Sweet, sour, salty, and bitter tastes	Sweet, bitter, astringent tastes	Hot, sour, astringent, and salty tastes
Bowel Movements	Irregular, inconsistent; tendency toward constipation; minimal or inconsistent reaction to laxatives	Frequent; tendency toward diarrhea; quick, strong reaction to laxatives	Slow, infrequent; moderate, consistent reaction to laxatives
Common Physical Challenges	Pelvic, lower body problems; sensitivity to pain; migrating pains; neuro-muscular and sensory issues	Mid-body problems; headaches; nausea; prone to inflammation	Above-the-neck problems; poor blood circulation; prone to metabolic problems

MENTAL CHARACTERISTICS

CHARACTERISTICS	WIND	FIRE	EARTH / WATER
Temperament	Nervous; physically, verbally, and mentally active; sensitive and responsive; changeable and inconsistent; impulsive; imaginative and creative; non-conformist; competitive, may bait others; enjoys socializing, laughing, and joking	Quick to anger, easily irritated; assertive; competitive and combative; highly motivated; compulsive; tendency toward obsessiveness and taking on too much responsibility	Relaxed, calm, gentle; dependable; stubborn and persevering; consistent, patient, tolerant, and long-suffering; lethargic; laconic, slow and monotonous; conformist, resistant to change
Emotions	Emotionally sensitive, reactive, unstable, and erratic; quick to move on and forgive; easily lonely, anxious, and afraid	Angry, hostile, jealous; impatient, proud, competitive; confident, egocentric; easily disgusted or indignant	Emotionally stable, nonreactive, unfazed; deep feelings of either contentment or sadness; slow to anger but slow to forgive; tendency towards depression
Confidence	Lack of self-confidence; unstable confidence	Very confident in own goals, knowledge, and abilities	Consistent, stable confidence but more modest, less performative
Mindset	Desirous, fearful	Focused on competition and business	Lazy, unbothered
Intellect	Agile, flexible; creative; selective intelligence; quick to learn, quick to forget; openness to novel ideas	Generally strong incisive intelligence; fast learners	Slow but steady learners; slow, deep thinkers
Memory	Good short-term memory; short attention span	Good long-term and short-term memory; clear, focused attention	Good long-term memory and retention
Socializing	Enjoys socializing, is balanced and soothed by socializing; highly sensitive to others' feelings and environment	Enjoys communal athletic and competitive activities	Builds relationships slowly and steadily
Common Mental Challenges	Anxiety; difficulty concentrating	Obsessiveness; anger management issues	Laziness, apathy; lack of mental clarity; confusion
Speech	Talkative; changes the subject often and easily	Precise, direct communication; quick responses; targeted responses or critiques that hit the mark	Less talkative; slower responses and longer pauses
Sleep	Light and interrupted; prone to insomnia; tendency to wake up before and around sunrise	Moderate amount of sleep; wakes up easily in the morning; tendency to wake up in hours around midnight	Heavy, deep sleeper; falls asleep easily, difficulty waking up
Dreams	Prone to unpleasant dreams and nightmares; fragmented, changeable, desirous, unsettled dreams; dreams of flying, moving, climbing	Bright, clear, vivid dreams; ego-focused or angry dreams; good dream recall	Simple, stable, calm, consistent dreams; extended dreams; otherwise, dreams might be hazy or minimal; less dream recall

health and longevity and the three fruits of a flexible mind, a sense of contentment, and overall happiness. And when you find what works for you, what balances and stabilizes you, just do that. Don't change because you encounter a new teacher or tradition. These days, marketing gives things sexy new names and makes us confused. Stay with what works for you in terms of food, herbs, exercise, and spiritual practice. It's individual. With that, let's turn to the typology self-assessment.

Typology Self-Assessment

To complete the typology self-assessment, you have two worksheets. The first is a Sowa Rigpa Typology Assessment. It is a chart of body and mind characteristics. For each characteristic, there are three choices— wind, fire, earth/water. You can read the descriptions and choose the element that best describes you. Then you have a second worksheet with a picture of a tree with three trunks—wind, fire, earth/water—and two branches per trunk—body and mind. So, for example, if you choose a body characteristic from the wind column, you then color a leaf on the wind-body branch that has a little fox at the end of it. If you choose a mind characteristic from the fire column, you then color a leaf on the fire-mind branch that has a little tiger at the end of it. After completing the assessment, you will be able to see your typology like a tree, showing you your elemental combination.

As you read the wind, fire, and earth/water descriptions for each characteristic, don't stress if you see yourself in two or even three of them. Just choose as many as you see fit and then color all of those leaves on the different branches. That said, it could be a sign of wind if you have difficulty making decisions. You don't have to be too precise. Your typology will reveal itself.

Of course, you can choose any colors you want for your leaves. You do you! But, traditionally, we use green/blue for wind, red/orange for fire, and gray for earth/water. At the end, you can also choose which animal feels like a match for your energy. Close your eyes and imagine yourself in a beautiful medicinal garden with gorgeous mountains, sweet sunshine, an uplifting breeze, and plentiful birdsong and animal calls. See yourself as an animal in the garden. Maybe you are a little fox, darting to and fro, keeping mystical secrets and also keeping an eye on everything, just in

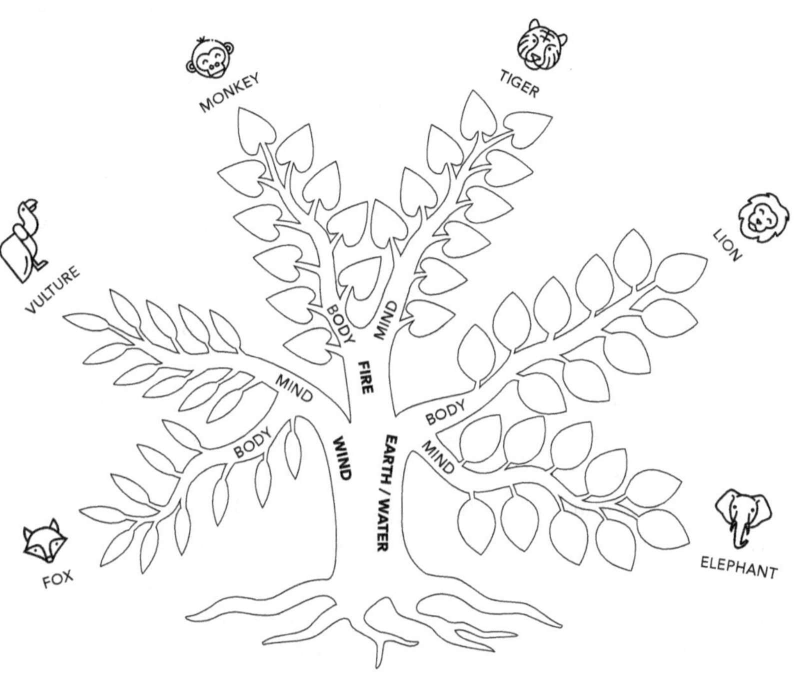

Typology coloring-in assessment exercise.

case. Or maybe you are a vulture, flying above, landing on a tree, looking around, and seeing what needs cleaning up. Or maybe you are a monkey, swinging from tree to tree with playful grace and not a moment to sit still. Or maybe you are a tiger, with a smooth walk, strong legs, and beautiful coat, ready to pounce at any moment. Or maybe you are an elephant, striding with a calm and steady presence, letting everything else get out of your way. Or maybe you are a lion with regal bearing, lying there and surveying the kingdom, leaving the action to your pride. Then try to imagine yourself as one of the elements. Maybe you are the breeze, gently animating the trees. Maybe you are the warmth of the sun, stimulating activity and growth. Maybe you are the water, flowing easily through the landscape. Maybe you are the earth itself, providing ground and stability. If you choose an animal or element that doesn't match the rest of your typology tree, then perhaps that animal and element are aspirational, showing you what you might need to balance your mind, energy, and body.

As you become more familiar with the elemental typologies, you might want to share this exercise with your family and friends. It can be a lighthearted way to get to know more about each other and even talk about habits and patterns that could be causing difficulties within your relationships. Similar to astrology, it gives us a framework to understand where others are coming from, and understanding builds compassion, patience, and equanimity. But, as with astrology, be careful not to use elemental typology to further construct stories of self. The purpose of these frameworks is not to drive us deeper into concepts of ourselves. Rather, they help us see the interdependence of elemental, environmental, and social influences in which we all play—and how to help the energy flow within and around us harmoniously.

These days, many of us live like gods, but we are actually hungry ghosts—craving, angry, insecure. We look outside of ourselves for peace and joy, going the wrong way toward superficial sources of temporary relief that ultimately bring us more trouble. It doesn't have to be like that. In the next three chapters, we are going to combine Yuthok's two treasures—the Yuthok Nyingthig and Sowa Rigpa—to create a program of healing across mind, body, and energy. You can consider it a program of spiritual health because it encompasses all aspects of your being. It is possible for you to feel happy, healthy, and whole—you just need the right medicine for your nature. Thankfully, you have now crossed paths with the gifted teacher and doctor Yuthok Yönten Gönpo. Whether you are excited about the idea of having a teacher or not, it doesn't matter. Yuthok said that: if you follow him, he will help you; if you don't follow him, he will help you; if you like him, he will help you; if you hate him, he will help you. True teachers don't care about fidelity or popularity. They care only about alleviating suffering—yours.

"You do not ignore your body
on the tantric path."

- Dr. Nida Chenagtsang

Chapter Three – Wind

Recall a time when you were alone in nature. You were sitting or walking. The air was still. All was still. Then a gentle breeze blew through. You saw tree branches sway, leaves dance a little. Maybe you heard the wind move through those branches and leaves, like they were talking to you. Maybe you saw their shadows glide across the ground. Maybe you became aware of your hair as it lifted. Maybe you felt your skin as it became cool. Maybe you caught the scent of nearby flowers or grass. Maybe you saw a bird play in the currents. Maybe you've even had the gift of watching a prayer flag lift, sending its wishes into the beyond.

Wind animates our world. It is the invisible force that makes everything feel alive. It helps us notice our sense experiences. It blows new views into the picture. It moves energy and matter around. When our wind element is balanced, we are playful and social. We bring levity to a situation and lighten the moment. We are creative and inventive. We come up with the fresh idea that changes everything. We are agile and flexible. We go with the flow and enjoy new experiences and embrace impermanence. We are intuitive and sensitive. We feel what is going on with self and other; we can read the room. We are compassionate and nurturing. We open our minds and hearts to really be there for others. Wind helps us love and laugh and celebrate the experience of being alive.

Similarly, in our physiology, wind energy helps our bodies flow. Our nervous system and our breathing depend on wind. The wind within the brain enables cognition, intelligence, and sensory functioning. It allows the mind to concentrate and retain information. Wind controls speech and enables us to swallow, salivate, and sneeze. It facilitates the psychological aspect of digestion, connecting brain with belly. It pervades the entire body helping us to contract and extend our limbs and also open and close our orifices. It enables the expulsion and retention of sexual and reproductive fluids, menses, feces, and urine. It empowers the dilation and contraction of the uterus and thus delivery during childbirth. Wind brought you into the world and helps you move through it—breathing, thinking, talking, walking.

When wind energy is imbalanced, we shift from dynamic to scattered. Even if you are not a wind type, you need to pay attention to wind imbalance because stress is wind. And we all have stress these days, so most of us have wind imbalance no matter what our typology. Also, wind dominates our later years—from 70 on—so it is easy to have wind imbalance as elders. Wind imbalance presents as excessive thinking. We are tossed around by thoughts, unable to land and focus. We change our minds easily, like we don't even know what to think. Our intuition and empathy turn into hypersensitivity and fragility. We are easily anxious and fearful about our lives, others' lives, the world at large. We become moody with erratic and unpredictable emotions. We are drawn to drama, stirring it up to get drunk on highs and lows. We talk a lot, saying many things, but not really making a point or even much sense. We seek chitchat and gossip, all part of the drama blah blah blah. We have a lot of social connections and relationships, but we struggle to maintain our boundaries and blow right through others. We can be hyperactive, running around without actually accomplishing anything. We do tasks fast, but miss the details. We fidget and can't sit still. Our excessive thinking and doing can turn into obsessive thinking and doing. We have recurrent fixations and repetitive actions. We might even turn that obsessive energy toward our bodies. We can't stop criticizing, fixing, or cleaning ourselves, looking for things that are wrong. We are the masters of negative self-talk, which amplifies our stress and anxiety. We might develop psychosomatic illnesses as the body reifies the brain's constant worrying. Our digestion and menstruation probably become irregular. Our skin feels dry and rough, our hair as well. We might have a cold feeling running through the body; we struggle to stay warm. Fingers and toes numb easily. We might have scattered pain, manifesting here and there without any clear physical or environmental cause. Our muscles become stiff and our tissues harden, and we lose flexibility in body and mind. We may be light-headed or dizzy or spacey at times. We could even dissociate, truly floating away, head in the clouds, lost in fantasies and fears, far from the grounded, embodied reality of here and now.

Accordingly, when your wind element is imbalanced, your primary mental toxin is desire. With your mind, energy, and body feeling frantic, you look outside of yourself for the answer. If you could just get that thing—the girl, the guy, the prize, the praise, the job, the house, the cash, the likes, the drink, the drug, the followers, the knowledge, the enlightenment—then you would feel better. Predictably, desire comes with a side dish of jealousy. Look at them over there with the thing. If you could have it, too, it would all be okay. The desire can be overt or subtle. But whenever you daydream about something other than right here, right now, desire is there. Desire is pervasive, like wind, blowing through your entire life, animating your imagination, kicking up your cravings, and pulling you away from the peace of presence.

When the poison is desire, what is the medicine? It is nourishment. Rather than looking outside of yourself for comfort, you nourish yourself within. This means nourishing yourself in body, energy, and mind. This means nourishing yourself in diet and lifestyle. This means nourishing yourself in spiritual practice. When you are nourished, you are balanced. And you feel whole—unto yourself. From that balance and wholeness, you can offer wind's uplifting activity to be of benefit to us all.

DIET AND LIFESTYLE

Here is the diet-and-lifestyle pith instruction for wind types: Put on your comfy clothes, snuggle into a sofa with a soft blanket, enjoy a cup of hot tea or warm soup, and have lighthearted, laughter-filled conversation with a loved one. Yum!

Wind types, and those with wind imbalance, thrive with a regular, relaxing lifestyle. For starters, you need to sleep eight to nine hours per night. This is your most important medicine of nourishment. You do well in warm and cozy places. The cold-plunge trend? No, no, no, not for wind types. For physical activity, try gentle sports, yoga, walking, and dancing. You can handle a mental or physical work life, but preferably only six or seven hours per day. Find some free time to spend with loved ones, and choose friends and lovers that feel nutritious. Spoiler alert, serious instruction on boundaries is coming. Also, pay attention to the content you take in such as music, media, and conversation—try to keep it all chill and relaxing. You can enjoy moderate amounts of sexual activity, partnered or solo. Another spoiler alert, we'll discuss Karmamudra, the yoga of bliss, later. An especially delicious medicine for wind is warm-oil massage. If you can get a warm-oil massage regularly, that would do wonders to balance your energy. You can also give yourself regular massages, with or without warm oil, especially on the crown of the head, center of the palms, and soles of the feet—the wind gates of the body. Heat up a little sesame oil, which is especially nourishing for wind, and see how a simple hand and foot massage can have the same effect as a day at the spa.

As part of your regular and relaxing lifestyle, wind types, and those with wind imbalance, need consistent meals. The fasting trend? No, no, no, not for wind types. Do not skip meals. Food is very grounding. You might scold yourself for emotional eating, but your intuition is right. You need to eat to ground yourself in your body. Just choose real food, rather than processed stuff, so you actually root and relax. This includes eating in a way that is rooting and relaxing—step away from stress and screens and sink into your meal. Wind is nourished by warm, oily, and nutritious food along with warm water and herbal teas. Warm milk, including plant based, can also be good for wind types. Vegetables that pacify and balance wind include onions and garlic (both are tranquilizers), pumpkin and carrots and squashes and potatoes and corn (think American Thanksgiving sides all day, every day), leeks and celery (lean like wind types), and seaweed and mushrooms (sea salty and earthy). Bananas, dates, figs, pears, watermelon, pomegranates, mulberries, and strawberries are good fruits for wind. Rice, millet, oats, quinoa, lentils, and beans are all great for wind. Oil is generally helpful for wind and especially ghee, butter, olive oil, and sesame oil. Yogurt and cheese, and plant-based dairy alternatives, are also good. Beef, chicken, fish, turkey, dried meat, and eggs are all good. Bone broth can be medicine for wind. The best spices for pacifying wind are salt, nutmeg, clove, cardamom, cumin, mustard, and coriander. A touch of sweetness is nice for wind as well.

But not too much sweetness. These days, everything seems to be extreme. When you were a teenager, doing extreme things with alcohol, drugs, music, and sex made sense as you were trying to explore edges and express yourself. But the problem is when you still do extremes as an adult. Something is nice, and you want to do it again and again. This is the path of addiction. All types struggle with addiction, but often it is wind energy fueling it—amplifying any elemental imbalance with the toxin of desire. A lot of us have addiction to sweets. Some say alcohol addiction is a sugar addiction as well. Hello, sweet humans. We say, "Home sweet home." Home is where we are supposed to receive love and connection and sweetness. But maybe home was bitter. Maybe mom was agitated and dad was aggressive. Don't blame them. They had problems because they had you. They had to worry about your future—schools, jobs, relationships, money. Worrying about these things is what parents and caregivers do, and then they get agitated and aggressive. When home sweet home is actually bitter, we look elsewhere to find that sweet taste. We seek out lovers to call "sweetheart." But maybe that relationship is bitter or spicy and not sweet. Our bodies might be craving the sweetness we can't find with others. Hello, sugar and alcohol. Instead of unsuccessfully nourishing yourself with an addiction to sugar and alcohol, you can truly nourish yourself through your spiritual path. You can rebuild a sweet emotional connection with yourself. Once you build that loving kindness and compassion toward yourself, you can send it out to others, even those where the connection has been bitter or spicy or bland.

SPIRITUAL PRACTICE

Now we will transition into spiritual medicine for wind. Maybe you have never thought of spirituality as something that could nourish you. But it can. We will look at Ngöndro practices, pre-empowerment practices, and post-empowerment practices of Guru Yoga/creation stage and completion stage—all with a focus on nourishing and balancing wind. Please note that what follows is a unique commentary on these practices. Of course, there is some instruction within the commentary. However, to practice Ngöndro, Guru Yoga, creation stage, and completion stage, you need a teacher to give you a reading transmission of the root text along with practice instructions. For now, you can explore the potential of these practices from the perspective of nourishing and balancing to consider how the Yuthok Nyingthig could help you be of benefit to yourself and others.

NGÖNDRO

Refuge

Releasing toxic desire, including addiction, begins here—by taking refuge in the Buddha as the doctor, Dharma as the medicine, and Sangha as the nurse. Until now, sweet windy one, you may have been looking for love in all the wrong places. Thanks to wrong view, we all go off course, driving ourselves toward the dead end of addiction, repeatedly taking refuge in any number of things, from drugs to phones to exercise to love dramas—all the way losing friends, lovers, money, stability, creativity, dignity, peace, joy, and, most of all, freedom. That can all stop now with the U-turn of refuge. When you find a reliable source of refuge, you have a deep feeling that you are now headed in the right direction. You feel a sense of protection—because you have found a true path, with real teachers and clear instructions, that brings proven results. You are safe now. You are going to learn how to be with any moment of mind and life that arises. You are going to learn how to handle anything. You are going to learn how to reclaim your confidence and creativity. You are going to learn how to be free—from the inside, no matter what is going on around you.

Taking refuge in the Buddha, Dharma, and Sangha is not magical thinking. It is not about flying off into space or indulging in make-believe. A lot of contemporary spirituality is ungrounded. You hear nice words about energy and love and spirits and all these things. But with that kind of talk, there is often no target. You are making a spiritual path with no goal. That is playing spiritual games, and that can be a problem. When you take refuge in the Buddha, Dharma, and Sangha, you know that this is not a game. There is a goal—to wake up. Waking up is the one clear solution to all of your problems. You need to wake up from this dream because it is actually a nightmare. The nightmare might look pretty, especially when it becomes a spiritual nightmare with cool clothes and exotic words and beautiful people. But it is still a nightmare of confusion, full of suffering. And no one is coming to save you.

So you need to wake up and find true freedom. You can do this by taking refuge in the Buddha, Dharma, and Sangha and dedicating yourself to evidence-based teachings and practices, supported by trusted teachers and a community of fellow practitioners. Once you take refuge, for real, you will feel you are on the right track. You will feel your suffering starting to diminish. You will feel your mind and life becoming easier. You will feel increasingly relaxed, safe, and secure. You will know you are on the right path. Your path will seem like an external path at first, but it is really an internal path—to your Buddhahood, the awakened Buddhahood within every being, waiting to be revealed. You will see how you can be nourished from within. In the Buddha, Dharma, and Sangha, you will have found a reliable source of refuge.

Bodhicitta

Oh, sweet windy one, you want to help. You have always wanted to help. You have loved ones you want to help, strangers you want to help, causes you want to help, an entire world you want to help. This is a good thing—to want to help. However, when we are not nourished from within, our attempts to help may be attempts to get help. Whether conscious of it or not, we believe that if we can help this person enough or that cause enough, then someone will give us the attention and security and love we seek. Again, you are looking for love in all the wrong places—outside of yourself.

It's okay. Somewhere along the way, you may have learned helping as a strategy to get love. True unconditional love does not need to be earned. But humans have a hard time unconditionally loving each other, until we are nourished from within. Before that, most of us love like a business transaction, sometimes overtly and sometimes subtly. So we all learn all kinds of strategies to get this business love from each other—and helping is a popular strategy, especially for empathic wind types. Of course, this helping strategy is conditional helping. It is business helping, just like business love—all wrapped up in attachment and desire. We are trying to get something from helping. Even if it seems generous and altruistic on the surface, underneath it can be shortsighted and self-centered—and even controlling and drama seeking. Ultimately, it brings self and other suffering. This unhelpful helping is an addiction of its own. Humans run in the hamster wheel of unhelpful helping all the time, even for entire lifetimes.

Now it is time to step out of the hamster wheel of unhelpful helping. You do not need to waste your precious mind and life on confused, conditioned strategies. You can use your natural empathy to learn how to really help. You can cultivate bodhicitta. You can make the aspiration to get enlightened for the benefit of all sentient beings. At the start of each and every practice, you can think about the loved ones you want to help, the strangers you want to help, the causes you want to help, the entire world you want to help—and you can dedicate your spiritual practice to all of it. Slowly slowly, you will see that you do not help people by getting overly involved in their lives; you help people by waking up and revealing your inherent Buddha Nature. A buddha knows exactly what is needed in every situation—what action or non-action will wake up everyone. This kind of compassionate action is the result of realizing the wisdom of emptiness and selflessness. Remember, the feminine principle of wisdom births the masculine principle of compassion. So the more you practice and wake up to your inherent wisdom, the more you will understand actual compassion and develop the skillful means to enact it. Keep contemplating and generating bodhicitta and let the practice do the work. You will develop a new understanding of the Six Perfections—generosity, morality, effort, patience, meditation, and wisdom. You will see a difference in the way you engage with others. You will settle down and quiet down and learn what really helps. And it will be such a relief for you.

The Four Immeasurables

The Four Immeasurables is also an opportunity to learn how to really help others. But, for starters, wind types need to learn how to help themselves, especially by setting boundaries, which helps everyone. The Four Immeasurables prayer in the Yuthok Nyingthig is a series of sentences that are spoken and contemplated:

> *May all beings have happiness and the causes of happiness.*
> *May all beings be free from suffering and the causes of suffering.*
> *May all beings never be separated from the supreme joy*
> *that is beyond all suffering.*
> *May all beings abide in equanimity, free from attachment,*
> *aversion, and sorrow.*

But often I tell people, especially wind types in need of nourishment, to start with you. After all, when you dedicate your practice to the benefit of all beings, you are included in these beings. So please begin the Four Immeasurables prayer making these wishes for yourself. Let these wishes land in your mind and body. Let them nourish you. It's good for you, and everyone, for you to be happy and joyful and steady and free from suffering. Honestly, we are all less trouble for each other when we feel content. So please begin the Four Immeasurables with this:

May I have happiness and the causes of happiness.
May I be free from suffering and the causes of suffering.
May I never be separated from the supreme joy
that is beyond all suffering.
May I abide in equanimity, free from attachment,
aversion, and sorrow.

After you make these wishes for yourself, you can repeat the prayer in the traditional way—using "all beings" instead of "I" and thinking of all the people you want to help. As with generating bodhicitta, this is a good opportunity to send your love to others and truly help them without getting all up in their business.

Additionally, wind types can be further nourished by a supplement to the Four Immeasurables. In earlier eras, this supplement was known as protection, but these days this supplement is known as boundaries. As mentioned, wind types often struggle with maintaining personal boundaries—and with respecting others' boundaries. Toxic desire and unhelpful helping can lead us into sticky situations—with friends, family, lovers, and strangers—that don't serve self or other. In order to cultivate loving kindness, compassion, joy, and equanimity for self and other, we all need to practice boundaries. Sweet windy one, you can keep people in your heart but please keep a healthy distance.

There is a traditional teaching on protection using five symbols of skillful means that can help with boundary setting. The first symbol is a wheel with eight spokes, and you visualize this wheel in your head. The eight spokes represent the Eightfold Noble Path. We have discussed right view with the Four U-Turn Thoughts and the Four Noble Truths.

From right view comes right motivation, right speech, right action, right livelihood, right effort, right mindfulness, and right concentration. As you align your life with the Eightfold Noble Path, you will develop the clean intention needed to cultivate safety for self and other in any connection. The second symbol is the lotus, and you visualize this lotus in your throat. When the lotus is in your throat, you speak clearly. You say what you want and don't want, what you can and can't do, what you will and won't do. If others don't like your choices, it is none of your business. As people, we have many different versions of ourselves. You have your version of you. Your friends have their version of you. Your exes have their version of you. Your parents have their version of you. People online have their version of you. With the lotus in your throat, you lose all desire to chase and manipulate and control other people's versions of you. Just speak your piece and that's that. The third symbol is the vajra, and you visualize this vajra in your heart. When the vajra is in your heart, you set a mental boundary. Remember the vajra is indestructible because it carries the wisdom of indivisibility. You know there are many causes and conditions for everything that happens. So it is ignorant and pointless to fixate on any one person or any single event or anything at all. You will never figure out them or why or any of it. You will just muddy your mind with incorrect theories because everyone and everything is complex beyond your imagination. So it is pointless to travel to the past and stir up memories or travel to the future and stir up fantasies. When thoughts arise to replay or revise or ruminate on some situation, you annihilate those thoughts with the vajra in your heart. In other words, don't even go there! With the vajra in your heart, you are secure and available for compassionate action in the present. The fourth symbol is the wish-fulfilling jewel, and you visualize this jewel in your navel. With this jewel, you know the difference between generosity and enabling. You know when and how to give. Moreover, you know that the best gift you can give anyone is the opportunity to wake up, and that won't happen if they are using you as a lifeline for anything at all. With the jewel in your navel, people will stop chasing you for this and that because you know when to offer support and when to say no more. The fifth symbol is the double vajra, and you visualize this double vajra in your genital region. While the single vajra sets the internal boundary of thought, the double vajra sets the external boundary of space. There are times when you need to completely cease contact with someone. You do this with people who want you to be their mama, who run after you to drink your milk, suck your blood, eat your bones. You do this with narcissistic people who pull you in with charm and then pull you under with control. It is a shock for all these people when you set the external boundary of space with the double vajra, when they can no longer influence and manipulate you. But it's good for them to lose you and good for you to lose them—because the problem is co-created. Use the double vajra to free you both. With this teaching on protection and boundaries, you have an active supplement to the Four Immeasurables. Over time, you will see how well they work together.

Prostrations

Prostrations can nourish wind types in several ways. First, prostrations can nourish you by building physical strength. Wind types may have trouble keeping weight on. Your body, like your mind, might feel all too ready to blow away in the breeze. Prostrations are a great workout. I have a friend who does three hundred prostrations every morning. People think he is a super-sporty gym guy. No, he just does prostrations. Prostrations work your entire body and help you feel safe and secure in your skin.

Second, prostrations can nourish you by building a healthy body image. Wind imbalance generates negative self-talk, especially blah blahs about your body. Through prostrations, you develop a different understanding of your body. Your body is no longer something for you to abuse or criticize. Your body is where you practice. Your body is your vessel for waking up. Your body is a precious opportunity. Through prostrations, you reroute your mind regarding your body.

Third, prostrations can nourish you by building confidence. Prostrations help you understand more and more how you can truly help self and other. When you prostrate, you visualize others prostrating with you—people you love, people you desire, people you fear, people you pity, anyone. Again, you will come to understand how to truly help these people, how to set appropriate boundaries, how to offer what is most beneficial in all situations. Invite others into your imagination as you prostrate and let the practice do the work.

Finally, prostrations can nourish you by building devotion. Prostrations create a connection with your teachers and your lineage. As you prostrate, you visualize Yuthok, or another guru, in front of you. With each prostration, you sow seeds of gratitude, growing a garden of devotion, nourishing your trust in your teachers and your path and your Buddhahood. Soon, you might find windy words are weeded out as the prostration prayer sprouts effortlessly:

> *From whose kindness great bliss itself instantly arises within us,*
> *the guru with jewel-like form, holder of the vajra,*
> *I prostrate at your feet.*

Mandala

Unfortunately, wind imbalance can inspire stinginess, neediness, and clinginess. Oh no! When we are worked up and windy, we feel ungrounded and thus unsafe and insecure. Enter toxic desire and attachment. We look to things and people for safety and security. And, once we get these things and people, we hold on to them. We grasp and grip. Not just physically but mentally. We won't let go. Out of windy instability, we even grasp and grip traumas and dramas, inviting them to haunt us like endless echoes.

Mandala practice can help you learn how to let things come and go. This will develop not only your generosity but also your equanimity. As you give visualized offerings to visualized teachers and buddhas, you ground yourself in the flow of life. Of course, you visualize precious objects and enjoyable experiences and offer them. But please allow difficult thoughts and painful feelings to surface and offer them as well. Good things and bad things, let it all arise, offer it up, and let it all dissolve. Over and over, you offer in this way while saying a prayer and repeating a mudra (hand gesture). Because this is only visualization, you are practicing feeling safe and secure as it all comes and goes—people, things, traumas, dramas. Moreover, you are offering this all to your compassionate teachers and buddhas. Because they are awakened, they have no preferences. You can lay whatever you like at their feet. They see it all as a glorious offering. Eventually, you will, too.

Circumambulation

Circumambulation combines three things that balance wind—gentle movement, a good friend, and a place to put your mind. Traditionally, circumambulations are performed by walking in a circle around a venerated object. In the Yuthok Nyingthig Ngöndro, you walk around an object representing Medicine Buddha. But, if possible, please go outside and take a walk. And please bring along all of those people you would like to help. See them all walking with you. Place your friend Medicine Buddha on your right shoulder and recite his mantra, audibly or silently— TADYATA OM BEKADZE BEKADZE MAHA BEKADZE RADZA SAMUDGATE SOHA. Mantra is a form of self-therapy. The word mantra means mind protection. You reroute your mind from fears and fantasies to sacred sounds. With practice, your mind will naturally flow to calming mantras instead of windy words. So please don't limit circumambulation to a formal practice. You can invite the safety and security of your friend Medicine Buddha, and the healing mantra, whenever you walk. Or run. Or stand in line. Or reach for your phone. The protection and support from Medicine Buddha and the mantra invite nourishment and relaxation for your nervous system. Medicine Buddha becomes a state of mind that shifts your way of being in the world.

Vajrasattva

Worry likes to ride on wind. For wind types, and those with wind imbalance, thoughts proliferate, especially thoughts of worry. You worry about your past—all the things that went wrong. You worry about your future—all the things that could go wrong. Worrying becomes your hamster wheel. Worrying becomes your confused refuge. But, with Vajrasattva, you can wash your worries away.

Please bring all of your worries to Vajrasattva. And let Vajrasattva's healing nectar drip down through your body and send your worries bye-bye. Remember Vajrasattva's energy is like a comforting hand, resting atop your head, calming you down. Let that feeling of comfort and calm flow through every bit of your body. You can see yourself as protected and resourced. You can trust that you know how to handle your life.

And don't stop with yourself. Sometimes wind imbalance creates what I lovingly call "grandma mind"—you worry about this person and that person and those people. Your first thought about anyone is to worry about them. Now, instead of worrying, you can visualize all of these people doing Vajrasattva practice with you and let healing nectar wash through them as well. You can see them as protected and resourced. You can trust that they know how to handle their lives.

I once had a dream where I had to cross a big river, very deep and strong. I thought, "Okay, I'm not good at swimming. It's difficult to cross this river. What will I do?" Then a yak came to help me. When I dream about yaks, they are protection dreams. This yak helped me cross the river. As I was riding this yak across the river, I thought, "This poor yak. He deserves some spiritual blessing." As soon as I had this thought, I saw Yuthok appear and dissolve into the yak's head. The yak was so happy to receive Yuthok's blessing. I then realized I was dreaming, but I thought, "This is good information. I know that if anyone needs Yuthok's blessing, I can imagine Yuthok is there above them and dissolves into them." When Yuthok dissolves into them, everything is transformed into great bliss.

So please don't reserve Vajrasattva for formal practice. Whenever you want to worry about someone, instead visualize Vajrasattva, or Yuthok or your favorite buddha or a ball of light, above their head and let healing nectar flow through them. Instead of sending negative worrying energy toward them or bothering them with your worries about them, you can think of them and be with them in a relaxed manner. Notice how your interactions and conversations with them become gentle and easy. And, of course, do this for yourself as well. Whenever you want to worry about yourself, instead visualize Vajrasattva, or Yuthok or your favorite buddha or a ball of light, above your head and let healing nectar flow through you. Instead of sending negative worrying energy toward yourself or bothering yourself with your worries about yourself, you can think of yourself and be with yourself in a relaxed manner. Notice how your interactions and conversations with yourself become gentle and easy.

Kusali Body Offering

Fear also rides on wind. The big fear is that something bad will happen to your body because your body is your biggest attachment—this is true for all of us. Remember the Buddha said the body is the ultimate troublemaker. And toxic attachment is the ultimate troublemaker for wind. So Chöd can be very helpful for wind types. As you cut, cut, cut your toxic attachment to your body, you free, free, free yourself from fear. People who practice Chöd become joyful—because they are free of fear. Chöd is like super duper mandala offering; you really learn how to let things come and go by letting your body come and go. Even better, instead of only offering to compassionate teachers and buddhas, you offer to a variety of guests—some you love, some you admire, some you avoid, some you fear. Bring them all to the feast. Let your body transform into whatever each one of them wants. Free from fear, you can give every being their perfect medicine. It's a preview for how it will be when you are enlightened. Your guests enjoy the feast and you are nourished by it.

PRE-EMPOWERMENT PRACTICE

Calm Abiding Meditation

Think of a time when you were outside on a windy day. Maybe tree branches and leaves were blowing around. Maybe your clothes got twisted and your hair got tangled. Maybe you couldn't hear or see well. Maybe you were rushing to get out of it all. Maybe you felt slightly panicked. And then you stepped inside. Maybe you let out a big exhale. Maybe you put down your things. Maybe you adjusted your clothes or changed into something warm. Maybe you brushed or untangled your hair. Maybe you made yourself a cup of tea and a snack. Maybe you sat down for a moment and rested. That calm abiding feeling with the exhale and the tea and the snack and the rest? That is what your mind can feel like when it comes in from the wind of your thoughts. Your mind can calmly abide.

Before you receive the Yuthok Nyingthig empowerment, you can practice calm abiding meditation. There are a lot of ways to practice calm abiding meditation. For wind types, and those with wind imbalance, it is very helpful to simply settle the mind. One way to do this is through sense experiences. Look at a nice flower or tree and let your mind rest on that object. Listen to beautiful music and let your mind rest on that sound. Eat something you enjoy and let your mind rest on that taste. Touch something warm and let your mind rest on that sensation. You can do these things for ten seconds or a minute or a few minutes. Come in from the windy thoughts and calmly abide. Do it whenever you remember to do it, maybe even a few times a day.

Once that practice is going well, you can create a practice of letting your mind rest on your breath. Using the breath as an object of focus is a tried-and-true meditation technique because your breath is always with you. Also, thoughts and breath move together. So the more you settle your breath, the more you settle your thoughts. To help settle your thoughts and breath, you can track the sensation of your inhales and exhales flowing in and out of your nose, or you can track the sensation of your ribs and/or belly expanding and contracting with your inhales and exhales. Or you can silently count your breaths. Inhale is one. Exhale is two. Inhale is three. Exhale is four. Count to ten and then start over. Know that many a meditator has found themselves at "sixty-four, sixty-five, oh shoot, I was supposed to start over at ten." Or you can silently say "in" and "out" with your breath. Inhale is in. Exhale is out. Or you can choose other words. If working with the breath feels uncomfortable, you can imagine a beautiful, natural object, like a flower or tree, in your heart center and let your mind rest there. Whatever technique you choose, you can place your body in whatever position is comfortable for you—sitting or lying down. You can set a timer for one to ten minutes, no longer than that. You can try this each day. And take it easy. Meditation is not a project; it is the release of projects.

But here is one key point. Inevitably, as you let your mind rest on an object of focus, your mind is going to float away over and over again. When you internally call your mind back to the object of focus, please use your gentlest voice. Think about how you would talk to a baby or a puppy. Use that voice. Meditation is a friendliness practice. You are becoming friends with your mind. So practice talking to yourself with kindness. Calm abiding—let it apply to your body, mind, and speech.

Three-Part Purification Breathing

Think about what you think about all the time. What is your top toxic attachment? What is your daily desire? Now imagine yourself as an animal going after that thing. Are you a bee buzzing around a mountain of sugary food? Are you a squirrel scrolling through your phone endlessly? Are you a tiger tracking your romantic interest? Choose an animal to represent this desire and attachment. Choose whatever you would like.

Then prepare to release that animal from your being and with it all of your desire and attachment. You can do this through a three-part breathing exercise. Take a smooth inhale, gently retain the breath for a moment, and on the exhale visualize a zillion of your attachment animals leaving the body through all of your orifices and pores. Bye-bye bees. See-ya squirrels. Ta-ta tigers. Smooth inhale, gentle retention, exhale the animals. If you want a sound to go with it, silently say "OM" on the inhale, "AH" on the retention, and "HUNG" on the exhale. If you want a color to go with it, visualize white light entering you on the inhale, red light spreading through you on the retention, and blue light leaving you with the animals on the exhale. Or choose other soothing sounds and colors. Or use the sounds and colors but not the animal visualization. Do it whenever you want or as a formal practice for a few minutes each day. Don't overthink it.

Mantra Healing

As mentioned, mantra, or mind protection, is a form of self-therapy. To nourish with mantra, keep it soft and slow. Say or sing mantras at a gentle pace that feels relaxing for you. Or you can play recordings of mantras and lie down, listen, and rest. A simple and powerful mantra is OM AH HUNG, which was suggested for the breathing exercise above. You can start there and see how it goes.

POST-EMPOWERMENT PRACTICE – CREATION STAGE

Outer Guru Yoga

Have people told you that you are too emotional? In your personal life or your work life, have people told you that it is problematic to be emotional? In your spiritual life and social life, have you felt shamed because you are emotional? Have you tried to shut down your emotions to fit in, stay cool, be chill? Have you felt exhausted by your emotions, like they take you on a rollercoaster ride or get you drunk and leave you hungover? Wind types, and those with wind imbalance, often have an abundance of emotions. Now, thanks to the genius of tantra, you can use your emotions to wake up. With Outer Guru Yoga, you can transform all of that emotional activity into devotional activity to help you feel nourished, stable, relaxed, and free.

Outer Guru Yoga is all about emotional connection. Through your human gratitude, humility, and vulnerability, you connect with your buddhas and teachers. Through their unconditional love and universal compassion, your buddhas and teachers connect you to the buddha and teacher within. It is brilliant spiritual technology.

You can do Outer Guru Yoga as a seven-day retreat and a daily practice. Either way, each time you begin a practice session, sit in a comfortable position and recite Refuge, Bodhicitta, and the Four Immeasurables. That will establish an altruistic motivation and good foundation for your practice.

Then, you visualize yourself as your buddha or deity of choice. Once you have received an empowerment, you can recreate yourself as a buddha or deity. Remember, with creation stage, you are recreating your moment of rebirth. At first this may sound odd and possibly incompatible with your worldview if you didn't grow up in a culture that posits reincarnation. But maybe think of it this way—you go through rebirth each morning when you get up. After the blackout of deep sleep and confusion of dreams, you arise as you and repeat your daily performance of you with all of your routine mental, energetic, and physical habits. Without the intervention of spiritual practice, that is what we do after we die. After the blackout of death and confusion of the bardo, we arise in a new form that is the embodiment of our routine habits, and then we continue playing them

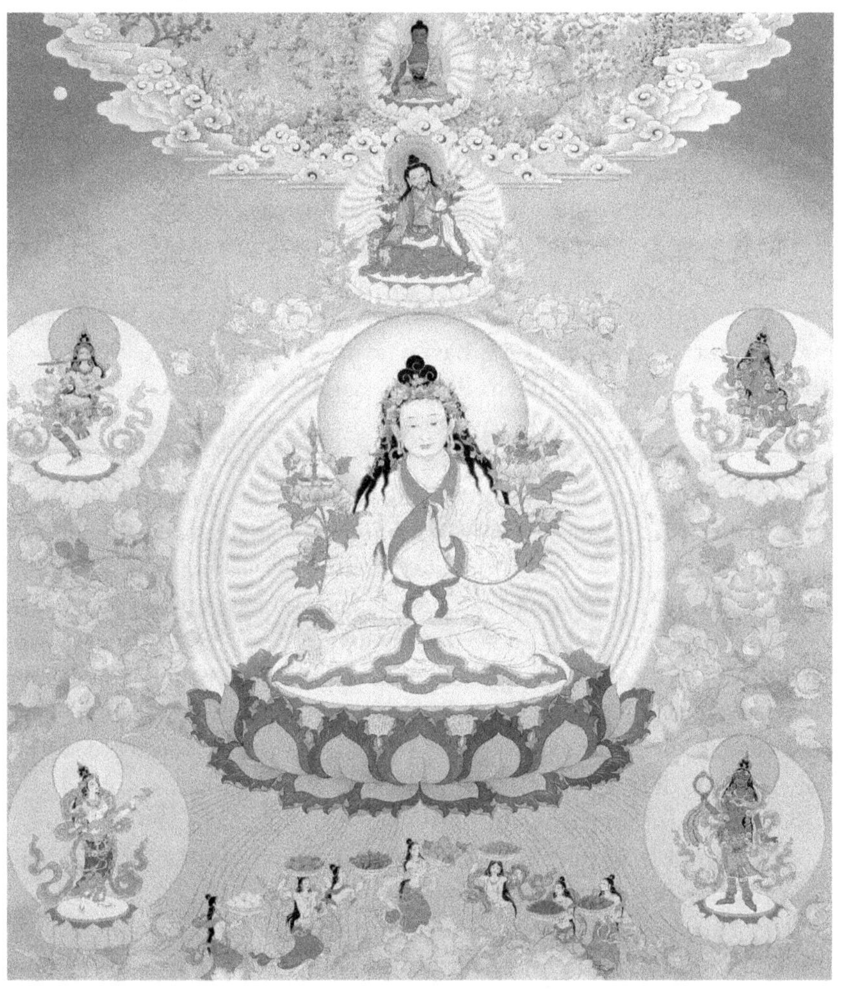

*Mandala with Yuthok in the center
surrounded by the four medicine goddesses.*

out. So, through the creation stage aspect of Outer Guru Yoga, you stop the habitual incarnation habit here and now, and instead recreate yourself consciously as a buddha to be of benefit to all beings—today and next life.

In Outer Guru Yoga, you are invited to recreate yourself as Medicine Buddha. This can be particularly helpful for balancing wind because Medicine Buddha is blue, and blue is a calming and healing color. Think about being the big blue sky in buddha form. It sounds nice, doesn't it? Also, Medicine Buddha heals all suffering, so you tap into an inner knowing of how to take good care of yourself. However, you don't have to generate as Medicine Buddha. Remember, Yuthok gives us freedom in creation stage practices. With many lineages, when you receive an empowerment, the text says you must generate as this or that buddha. But what if you already have a favorite buddha for creation stage? Then you feel like you have to divorce that old buddha and marry this new buddha. Sometimes we divorce too many buddhas and then have a string of jilted buddhas trailing after us. So if you already feel married to a buddha or deity, be it male or female, peaceful or wrathful, please stay with that buddha or deity. Familiarity and consistency can also balance wind. If you don't have a buddha or deity, then generate as Medicine Buddha and let the healing blue light permeate your form. If you have clear visualization, that is good. But if you don't have clear visualization, don't worry. Focus on feeling yourself as a three-dimensional, blue-light body, empty of bones and organs, like a hologram. Your head is blue light, your hair is blue light, your neck is blue light, your arms are blue light, your chest is blue light, your belly is blue light, your back is blue light, your genitals are blue light, your legs are blue light, your skin is blue light. Take your time to physically and emotionally feel yourself as healing blue light. You are practicing being a buddha.

Then you build your connections. When you were born in this life, you had people all around you, like family and their friends. So now you are consciously choosing connections to support your rebirth as a buddha. To begin, there is your enlightened guru, Yuthok, sitting on a four-petaled pink lotus above your head. He is also made of light. He is wearing a white robe, and he has flowers in his long black hair. In his right hand, he is holding a blue utpala flower that contains a text and a sword, representing the feminine principle of wisdom and emptiness. In his left hand, he is holding a pink lotus that contains a vase and a vajra, representing the masculine principle of compassionate action.

You visualize Yuthok above your head because this is the location of the crown chakra. Right now, we don't physically have anything here, but energetically we all have a thousand-petaled lotus waiting to open. You often see buddhas depicted with a topknot of hair because when you become a buddha the chakra in your forehead rises and becomes a protrusion on top of the head. Don't worry about having a bump on your head as a buddha; you, too, can cover it with a cool topknot hairdo. For now, visualizing Yuthok on top of your head allows you to feel this powerful crown chakra waiting to open. And, again, if you already have a guru other than Yuthok, that is fine. Maybe you have a wrathful guru or a female guru or a wrathful female guru. Or maybe you try to see Yuthok in a white robe, but you see him in a yellow robe. Or maybe you see Medicine Buddha above your head instead of Yuthok. You don't need to say, "Go away, Medicine Buddha! I need Yuthok here!" Whatever you see, it is all good. They are all one in nature. Yuthok is a bridge to all gurus.

In fact, through Yuthok, you call in all the buddhas, deities, and teachers that resonate with you. You imagine light radiating from visualized Yuthok's head, throat, and heart chakras out into the universe. This invites the real Yuthok. Because Yuthok attained the rainbow body, his body is now light and pervades all time and space. When you call him, he comes to you. He dissolves into the visualized Yuthok above your head like water adding to water. Do not doubt this. Yuthok said that he will appear to whoever calls him. And he brings all the gurus who are meaningful for you. Whoever you believe in, whoever is your spiritual guide, whoever is your enlightenment role model, whoever is your protector, all of these beings dissolve into Yuthok. Let Yuthok be the representative of all these gurus. Let them be all in one with no separation. Let yourself feel gratitude, humility, and vulnerability in the face of all these gurus who are here for you. Let yourself feel safe and secure knowing all your gurus are always with you.

Please remember to include your human teachers that you know and love. Be emotional. Be devotional. Yuthok is the bridge to all of your human teachers. Feel their indivisibility with Yuthok. Feel their presence with you. Feel their complete acceptance of you. Feel their love for you exactly as you are. In fact, it is even more important to feel your human teachers with you than any buddhas or deities. There is a nice story about Guru Rinpoche that makes this point. Guru Rinpoche is considered to be the founder of Tibetan Buddhism because he brought the teachings successfully to Tibet from India. One time, he was meditating with his students, and he generated a huge wrathful deity right next to him. His students could see the deity and were wowed by this beautiful being of light. Then Guru Rinpoche asked his students if they wanted to receive the empowerment from the deity or him. Almost all of his students said that they wanted to receive the empowerment from the deity; they said that now the deity was here they didn't need the teacher. But Guru Rinpoche's main student, a woman named Yeshe Tsogyal, said the deity was a manifestation of her teacher, so she wanted to receive the empowerment from her teacher. Then the deity dissolved into Guru Rinpoche. So the ones who wanted to receive the empowerment from the deity didn't receive the empowerment. Because of her devotion to her teacher, Yeshe Tsogyal received the empowerment from Guru Rinpoche. I like this story. Because for me, in my practice, I visualize Yuthok and all the buddhas, but once I think of my Yuthok Nyingthig teacher, Khenpo Troru Tsenam, dissolving into Yuthok, then emotionally it becomes very personal and powerful. Try it and see for yourself. With Outer Guru Yoga, it is essential to feel this personal and emotional connection.

In the visualization above your head, Yuthok is surrounded by four medicine goddesses. Again, you had many people around you when you were born, like relatives and siblings. Now, as you consciously recreate as a buddha, you are supported by four medicine goddesses or deities of any gender and form you would like. The four medicine goddesses represent the four tantric activities, and they help you with your worldly life. In front of Yuthok, to the east, is the white goddess. She plays a lute. She is the pacifying goddess. You can ask her to pacify illness, conflicts, anxiety, stress, anything that needs calming for you or your loved ones or the world. To Yuthok's right, to the south, is the yellow goddess. She plays a flute. She is the increasing goddess. You can ask her to increase material wealth, work opportunities, memory, intelligence, generosity, strength, sleep, energy, anything that needs increasing for you or your loved ones or the world. Behind Yuthok, to the west, is the red goddess. She plays a trumpet. She is the magnetizing or controlling goddess. You can ask her to magnetize or control anything in relationships, work, family, behavior, emotions for you or your loved ones or the world. To Yuthok's left, to the north, is the green goddess. She holds a silver mirror. She is the destroying goddess. You can ask her to destroy any obstacles and negative energy affecting you or your loved ones or the world. She is particularly good at destroying outer, inner, and secret obstacles to your spiritual practice.

Out of gratitude for their love and support, you offer visualized mandalas, flowers, and music to Yuthok and the four goddesses. Offer whatever beautiful objects mean the most to you. All of those attachments you have? Now is your chance to give them as an offering. Then offer the sense pleasures that mean the most to you. All of those desires you have? Now is your chance to give them as an offering. Then offer whatever fruits of your practice mean the most to you. All of that equanimity, joy, and bliss? Now is your chance to give this as an offering.

Having offered from your heart, you can then ask the four goddesses to help you with specific aspects of your life through their activities of pacifying, increasing, magnetizing/controlling, and destroying. I like this aspect of Outer Guru Yoga because sometimes we try to meditate, but we are worried about people who are sick. Then we ask the white goddess to heal them. Or we are worried about money. Then we ask the yellow goddess to increase our work opportunities. Whatever ordinary wishes you have, these goddesses will fulfill them. Please do not be shy. They want to help. Ask them for assistance at the start of practice so your mind can settle down. Trust that they can make your ordinary life as you would like it to be.

But even if your ordinary life is perfect, one thing is still missing—spiritual enlightenment. You ask Yuthok to help you with that. Let all of your emotion and devotion flow. You cannot wake up on your own. You need the help of the Buddha, Dharma, and Sangha. Please ask for it. In response to your heartfelt request, Yuthok again radiates light to collect the blessings of all the buddhas and to bless all sentient beings. The blessings return as light and condense into the vase in Yuthok's left hand. Then the vase overflows with blessings and drips healing nectar into your crown point on the top of your head. Like Vajrasattva practice, this healing nectar flows as liquid or light throughout your entire body.

As the nectar flows through each of your chakras—head, throat, heart, navel, base—you receive the empowerments that you received when your teacher gave you the empowerment to do these practices. In this way, Outer Guru Yoga is a self-empowerment practice. You have consciously recreated as a buddha, and now you are re-empowering yourself with the body, speech, mind, qualities, and activities of all the buddhas.

As you receive the healing nectar and empowerments, there is a mantra for you to say, audibly or silently—OM AH HUNG MAHA GURU GUNA SARVA SIDDHI HUNG DZA DEVA DAKINI HARINISA TSITA HRING HRING SAMAYA DZA HUNG BAM HO. With this mantra, you are asking Yuthok to bless your body, speech, and mind with the blessings of all buddhas and to transmit to you all the common spiritual powers (skills that help you help others) and uncommon spiritual powers (enlightenment); you are also asking all the male and female buddhas and the four medicine goddesses to bless you with their hearts and commitments so that all universal healing energy dissolves into you. You call out with your heartfelt yearning for Yuthok's promised speedy blessing. If you are musical, you can make a nice tune and sing this mantra over and over again. You can even record it to play as you practice. As you say the mantra and visualize the healing nectar, you are filled with the blessings of all buddhas, gurus, teachers, goddesses, and healers. These blessings fill you completely. Imagine and feel the nectar all throughout your light body. You are free from ordinary thoughts and confusion and suffering. Everything becomes blissful.

When you feel complete, the four medicine goddesses dissolve into Yuthok, and Yuthok dissolves into your heart. Then your visualized form of Medicine Buddha dissolves into Yuthok at your heart, and Yuthok dissolves into space. Rest in that space. When you are ready, you then arise from your practice with no separation between you and Yuthok, between you and all buddhas and deities, between you and all your teachers and gurus. You are completely recreated as a buddha. You are healed, loved, whole, joyful, safe, and nourished from within. You are wise and compassionate and eager to be of benefit. You are ready to do your day as a display of your inherent Buddha Nature and to see everyone else as a display of their inherent Buddha Nature.

Outer Guru Yoga is a creative spiritual way to build confidence, which is important for balancing wind. If we try to build confidence in mundane ways, it gets blocked by our fixation on I and self. We aim for self-confidence but end up self-conscious and self-centered. This can even happen with meditation practice. Oh, I am meditating. Oh, I am a special meditator. Because of self-attachment, many spiritual things become another avenue for building stories about I and self. It is better to put our pure vision into the guru, Yuthok, and his perfect blessings, and then dissolve his blessings into us and see the perfection in ourselves and everything. It is an interesting and effective psychological approach to understanding and displaying our Buddha Nature and recognizing everyone else's Buddha Nature—and this is true confidence. Fortunately, wind types all well suited for this wind-balancing practice. Wind types often have lots of fantasies and feelings. Bring them all to this practice. Let your emotion and devotion create an imaginative scene that serves your awakening.

As you do this practice again and again, you will build a deep connection to Yuthok and your teachers. Once you have this connection, you will spiritually expand. All the other practices will become easy for you. Outer Guru Yoga is extremely powerful, and it is the heart of Tantric Buddhism.

POST-EMPOWERMENT PRACTICE – COMPLETION STAGE

Illusory Body Yoga

What happens when someone says something good about you? You are happy. Oh, this person is saying good things about me; I'm so happy! Maybe you even say good things about that person. It is a happy day. What if that same person says something bad about you? You are unhappy. Oh, this person is saying bad things about me; I'm so unhappy! Maybe you even say bad things about that person. It is an unhappy day.

What happens when you get what you want? You are happy. Oh, I got what I want; I'm so happy! Maybe you want to help others get what they want. It is a happy day. What if you don't get what you want? You are unhappy. Oh, I didn't get what I want; I'm so unhappy! Maybe you don't want to help others get what they want. It is an unhappy day.

Good. Bad. Happy. Unhappy. Up. Down. Your emotions swing back and forth. This affects how you see the world. This affects what you say to others. This affects how you behave. You are like a puppet—waiting for others' words to tell you how to feel, think, speak, and act. You are like a toy—waiting for life circumstances to tell you how to feel, think, speak, and act. You are not free. You are not free at all.

Don't blame others. Don't blame life. You have made yourself a puppet and a toy. It's worse than that. You have made yourself a prisoner—a prisoner of your mind. Only you can do that to you. Only you can make yourself a puppet, a toy, a prisoner. This is good news. Because this means you can liberate yourself. You do not need to rely on anyone else for this. You can and must self-liberate. Because when your mind is free, you are free—no matter what somebody says to you, no matter what life throws at you. Even if you ended up in a physical prison, you would be free because your mind is free. Mind frees itself by uncovering its true nature of bliss. But you have to work through waves of emotions to get there. You have to swim out past the choppy breakers to float in the vast ocean of love, compassion, joy, and equanimity.

One way to make it through the emotional breakers is Illusory Body Yoga. Illusory Body Yoga is like Buddhist self-therapy. It defuses the power of the Eight Worldly Concerns—praise and blame, success and failure, pleasure and pain, fame and disgrace—to release you from the highs and lows of emotions. And you do this by coming to know the truth of your body—the biggest troublemaker of self-attachment.

As you will come to understand more and more, your body is an illusory body. You actually have a lot of illusory bodies. You have this physical body that you identify with most. You also have a body in the mirror's reflection. You also have a body in your dreams. You also have a body in your thoughts and fantasies. You also have many other bodies in others' dreams, thoughts, and fantasies about you. You also have an energetic body that you are experiencing through creation stage practice. But you mostly get stuck with the physical body because you identify that one with yourself. You get stuck thinking about yourself, so you get stuck thinking about this physical body and its experiences. You want to receive praise but not blame in this body. You want to have success but not failure in this body. You want to have pleasure but not pain in this body. You want to have fame but not disgrace in this body. You want or don't want all these things to happen in this physical body that you identify with yourself. So you get stuck thinking about your beauty, skin, hair, weight, wrinkles, and age. You get stuck thinking about being good, smart, popular, funny, talented, and sexy. You get stuck thinking about having the right relationship, job, money, house, car, and travel. You get stuck thinking about experiencing the best kiss, touch, and sex. Then you get stuck being a puppet and a toy as you hear what you want or don't want, get what you want or don't want, experience what you want or don't want—and have emotional swings because of it all.

You start to feel so tired, tired of your life, tired of everything. You know why you feel tired? Because you are swinging between hope and fear. You are chasing praise, success, pleasure, and fame and you are running from blame, failure, pain, and disgrace—within this body. In this society, you need to do so many superficial and artificial things because of these Eight Worldly Concerns. In fact, driven by the hope and fear of these concerns, we have created a society that is superficial and artificial. So you get all dolled up in your superficial puppet outfit and artificial toy clothes as you chase praise, success, pleasure, and fame and run from blame, failure, pain, and disgrace. At the end, you don't even know who or what you truly are. That is why tantra instructs you to recreate yourself as the buddha you truly are. Now, having that insight and power through creation stage practice, you can free yourself from the superficial and artificial prison of the Eight Worldly Concerns through the completion stage practice of Illusory Body Yoga.

Illusory Body Yoga is especially nourishing and beneficial for wind types who tend to be quite sensitive and easily caught up in the mental whirlwind of hope and fear. Sweet windy one, your sensitivity is a strength. As we have discussed, wind types are perceptive, empathic, devotional, vulnerable, and eager to help our world—all qualities that rise to the top of humanity because of wind. However, wind imbalance blows that sensitivity into fragility. When our wind is imbalanced, we take things very personally, and we feel extreme highs and lows. Our emotional dramas become an addiction of their own—one that everyone around us gets swept into. Rather than bringing the lightness of wind to a situation, we suck all the air out of a room. But you can free yourself, and others, from painful emotional cycles with Illusory Body Yoga. Those blustery, moody waves that you mistake for you? Those waves can subside, and you, too, can float in the vast blissful ocean of mind's true nature.

Illusory Body Yoga is an easy practice in terms of form. It has two steps—impure Illusory Body Yoga and pure Illusory Body Yoga. Traditionally, you stay in retreat for seven days to do Illusory Body Yoga. You make a decision to be done with emotional highs and lows, and you dedicate a week to do so. If you can't do retreat, you can do Illusory Body Yoga as a daily practice for an extended period of time. Either way, you always start with Guru Yoga. You ask for help and blessings from Yuthok and all the buddhas and lineage teachers you would like to invite. Though you have to do this work yourself, you cannot do it alone. Like all who have become enlightened, you need the support of buddhas, gurus, teachers, and lineage to help you fearlessly free yourself.

You start with impure Illusory Body Yoga. To do this, first list the five things you most want to hear. You want to hear these things from your parents, your partners, your lovers, your children, your friends, your colleagues, the online masses. You want so much to hear these things. But you don't hear them. So you are struggling. What are these things? Maybe… you are beautiful, you are kind, you are smart, you are talented, you are authentic, you are special, you are the best. Think deeply about your list of five things you want to hear. Then sit in front of a mirror, look at your reflection, and say the first phrase to yourself five times. Say it slowly and with meaning. You are so beautiful. You are so beautiful. You are so beautiful. You are so beautiful. You are so beautiful. Pause. Then say the next phrase to yourself five times. After you finish saying all of these phrases, look at your reaction in the mirror.

Next, list the five things you do not want to hear. Maybe… you are a failure, you're so freaking ugly, nobody likes you, I'm so disappointed in you, you are getting old, you will never be loved. Again, look at your reflection and say each phrase slowly five times. Look at your reaction in the mirror.

Next, imagine that other people respect you. Look at your reflection and imagine many admiring people all around you. Maybe all of your colleagues are complimenting you. Maybe you are a teacher and all of your students love you. Maybe you are on a podcast and all of the listeners are impressed by you. Maybe you are posting beautiful images of yourself online, and everyone thinks you are gorgeous and wants to be you. Maybe your parents are praising you. Maybe your children are honoring you. Maybe your spouse, partner, lover adores you. Maybe others desire you. You can say these things to your reflection as you imagine your dreams and wishes coming true. Look at your reaction in the mirror.

Next, imagine that nobody respects you. Look at your reflection and imagine there is nobody admiring you at all. Maybe your colleagues are talking about your stupidity behind your back. Maybe your students are rolling their eyes and finding other teachers. Maybe you are shunned for your remarks on that podcast. Maybe you post pictures online, and most people don't care and others gossip about how bad you look. Maybe your parents are disappointed in you. Maybe your children think you are a loser. Maybe your spouse, partner, lover ignores you. Maybe you are not desired by anyone. You can say these things to your reflection as you imagine all you dread is happening. Look at your reaction in the mirror.

Next, imagine you have everything you want in life. What do you want in life? Don't just say enlightenment. There are so many other things you want in your life. Think about all the things you want, how you would live in a different way if you had them. Whatever it is, it's okay. Don't judge. Just imagine it all and tell your reflection that you have everything you want. Look at your reaction in the mirror.

Next, imagine you don't have anything you want. More than that, you lose everything you have. Maybe you lose your phone, your computer, your clothes, your car, your home. Maybe you lose your friends, your family, your colleagues, your lovers. Everything and everyone is gone from your life. Imagine this and tell your reflection that you have lost everything. Look at your reaction in the mirror.

Next, imagine you are experiencing great pleasure. Maybe you experience the best massage, tantric massage, Thai massage, foot massage, herbal baths, the most exquisite kiss, the most erotic touch, the sexiest sex. Imagine the delicious things you want to experience. Tell your reflection you are experiencing these delightful things. Look at your reaction in the mirror.

Next, imagine you are experiencing great pain. Maybe you are chased, you are beaten, you are even killed. Imagine the horrors you do not want to experience. Tell your reflection you are experiencing these awful things. Look at your reaction in the mirror.

With all of this, what is the reaction of your reflection in the mirror? It's kind of bored, isn't it? You say these good things; you say these bad things. You imagine these wonderful things; you imagine these terrible things. Maybe internally you are feeling joy or feeling sorrow. But your reflection in the mirror is unfazed. It is similar to when you have a stressful dream. Maybe you have had the dream where you are naked in front of people. It is a very intense dream. You feel shame and panic. You are terrified that people will see your genitals. You try to cover your front. You try to cover your back. You try to cover both. You don't know how to move. You come up with this and that strategy. You think you are so smart with your strategies to get out of this naked situation. But when you wake up, you see you were being so stupid. You were stressed out for no reason; it was just a dream. Your dream body was confused and upset; but your physical body was the smart one, still resting during the dream. With Illusory Body Yoga, your physical body is now the confused one, experiencing emotional highs and lows. Not to mention your thought-and-fantasy body is totally out of control, running here and there, as you contemplate all these scenarios. So your reflection body is now the smart one. Your reflection body is present. Your reflection body is not having a big reaction. Your reflection body is not a puppet or a toy. Your reflection body is free of emotions entirely. Your reflection body displays equanimity. Your reflection body is now your guru.

Impure Illusory Body Yoga is like allergy prevention. Many little kids have an egg allergy, and the best recipe for an egg allergy is egg itself. You give them a little egg for one month. The next month, you give them a little more. Slowly slowly, they will become free from this egg allergy. You can do the same with your emotions. Don't push yourself too much in the beginning, especially with the negative things—the mean words, the disrespect, the loss, the pain. These things trigger you because you are scared they are going to happen or they have happened already. You have an allergy to these things. So you can use this meditation in a mild and gradual way. You give yourself some emotions; you give yourself a little more. Slowly slowly, you will become free from emotional allergies. You will be immune to these words and these scenarios. Like your guru in the mirror, you will be unfazed. We have a Tibetan proverb that says words are invisible but they can scar somebody's mind and heart. With impure

Illusory Body Yoga, your mind and heart become invincible to invisible words. You will still have emotions; you are human. But you will be free of hope and fear, the big ups and downs, the choppy breakers that toss you around. You will know how to float in the vast ocean of mind, letting waves come and letting waves go.

Keep returning to the Buddha's enlightenment story. There is deep teaching in those moments when the maras were trying to sabotage the Buddha's liberation. They were shooting arrows and spears; they were offering sensual delights. But the Buddha was just sitting, like your reflection in the mirror, because he knew that the maras were illusory. He also knew that these illusory maras were scared of being revealed as superficial and artificial, just like the Eight Worldly Concerns. In the face of the Buddha's powerful, awakened energy, these illusory maras were prideful, jealous, desirous, angry, and confused, just like the stories of I and self. In his wisdom of emptiness, the Buddha knew that the compassionate way to defeat the illusory and toxic maras was not to fight back and play their game. Instead, he displayed patience and equanimity. Fearlessly, he watched the maras' weapons and temptations come at him and then turn into flowers. Over and over again, the weapons and temptations came at him and then turned into flowers. It took a long time for the maras to lay down their weapons and temptations. But they did. Because the Buddha saw the maras and their weapons and temptations for what they truly are—energy, vibration, sound, light. It was all just impermanent waves in the ocean, maybe even beautiful in their motion.

After practicing impure Illusory Body Yoga, you may naturally fall into pure Illusory Body Yoga. Like your reflection in the mirror, you will be bored by the good words and the bad words, the wonderful scenarios and the terrible scenarios. You will relax. With your reflection body relaxed and your physical body relaxed and your thought-and-fantasy body relaxed, you are free from the distractions of I and self; you are free of the Eight Worldly Concerns. In this state, you can more easily feel your energy body, an overall awareness and aliveness, a spacious presence, maybe even an ocean of bliss. You are sensing the buddha within you, which you generate during creation stage practice. If it helps, in pure Illusory Body Yoga, you can consciously generate yourself as a being of light—either in your form or in the form of a buddha or deity. The most important aspect of the practice is experiencing this uncreated and indestructible presence within you. With completion stage practice, you realize this presence is always here, waiting to be of benefit to you and others.

Slowly slowly, you will see and know the illusory nature of all these bodies of yours. The physical body, the reflection body, the dream body, the thought-and-fantasy body, even the energy body—they are all an ever-changing display of causes and conditions. None of them have any ultimate solidity or reality. Just because you identify with one more than another, at any given moment, it doesn't make that body more real, or real at all. You will feel how you are bigger than bodies. You are beyond space and time, transcendent, all pervasive, like a rainbow, at once appearing and empty, like Yuthok, like everything.

Karmamudra

Let's cut to the chase. Karmamudra involves sexuality. In the West, many people think tantra is all about sex, but this is a big misunderstanding. Sexual practice can be included in Tantric Buddhism—or not. Through this book, I hope you see the wide range of practices offered in Tantric Buddhism, particularly in the Yuthok Nyingthig. There are 84,000 poisons, and there are 84,000 medicines. So if you have distracting desire, sexual or otherwise, Karmamudra could be just what the doctor ordered to transform your toxic attachment into brilliant bliss.

Of course, most humans do have sexual desire at some point in their lives, but I am introducing Karmamudra here for wind types because desire is the poison most stirred up by wind imbalance. And, of course, people other than wind types can have wind imbalance. All to say, Karmamudra is available for anyone who is interested in transforming mundane desire into spiritual liberation. Anyone of any sexuality, any sexual orientation, any sex, any gender, any body, you are welcome to practice Karmamudra. Anyone with sexual partners and anyone without sexual partners, you are welcome to practice Karmamudra. Anyone at all, you are welcome to practice Karmamudra. That said, to practice Karmamudra, you need to receive transmission and instructions from a qualified teacher. So, in this book, I will only provide a brief introduction to the practice. I have an entire book written about Karmamudra, entitled *Karmamudra: The Yoga of Bliss*, which I wrote in part to clear up misunderstandings about tantra and to help prevent sexual abuse. If you are interested in pursuing Karmamudra further, maybe look at that book, say a prayer that you encounter a teacher to give you these teachings, seek out the proper empowerment, and set about practicing Ngöndro as well as Guru Yoga. For now, know that you do not need to shut down or shame your sexual desire on the Tantric Buddhist path. Just the opposite—you can celebrate your sexuality as a powerful energy that can lead you to awakening.

And how does Karmamudra do that? Through increasing bodhicitta. When we talk about Karmamudra, we must talk about bodhicitta. Then there is no bullshit. Otherwise, there is blah blah about sex and energy, and the bull of bullshit gets very big. It is important to understand that the essence of Karmamudra is bodhicitta. That's it.

We talked about bodhicitta in Ngöndro—it is the mind that is focused on benefiting others. With Karmamudra, we explore the energetic mechanics of developing this altruistic and compassionate mind. There are two levels of bodhicitta energy. The first is relative bodhicitta, which is the felt experience of love in all its forms—romantic love, familial love, loving kindness—that inspires us to be of benefit to others. An easy way to think of relative bodhicitta is the happy hormones that arise during any loving connection. For many people, romantic love and sexual desire are the quickest and strongest shortcuts to these happy hormones. Think about the first day you are in love with someone. It is not just your new lover but the entire world that is lovely. Think about your orgasm. It is not just super pleasure but super duper pleasure. With Karmamudra, you can learn how to increase and sustain those happy hormones through the efficient energetic and neural pathways that are usually only used by romantic love and sexual desire. In so doing, you expand your altruism and compassion beyond romantic lovers and family members to more and more beings.

There are a variety of practices within Karmamudra that can do this. There are mindful, blissful breathing practices that you can do on your own or with a partner. There are mindful, blissful sexual practices that you can do on your own or with a partner. Basically, you learn how to activate the happy hormones of relative bodhicitta whenever you so choose. For example, you could allow yourself to be awash in joy just from inhaling and exhaling. As you increase your moments of pleasure in life, you decrease your moments of suffering. The brain and body can only do one thing at a time—and no one is thinking about their to-do lists, let alone their traumas and dramas, during orgasm. So, through Karmamudra, you are training your mind, body, and energy to reorient toward bliss, which is your natural state. And, again, that natural state of bliss inspires an increase in altruism and compassion toward others.

But, please understand, becoming a Karmamudra practitioner does not mean you are whiling away your days dramatically deep breathing and moaning in delight. This practice is a means to an end—revealing your natural mental, physical, and energetic baseline of wholeness and aliveness. This means you feel good just being. You feel so good just being that you stop anxiously chasing after others to fill some unfillable hole of need. Hello, windy people? You can still enjoy romantic relationships, if you would like, but your connection will come from sharing mutual wholeness and aliveness. Further, once you stop chasing, broadly speaking, you can focus on being of benefit. On that note, through Karmamudra, the pure view of creation stage comes easier. You fall in love with the world. And, when you are in love with the world, you will stop causing trouble for the world by trying to seduce the world, reject the world, sell the world, buy the world, fool the world, shoot the world. You will quietly lose interest in anything other than simply loving the world and benefiting its beings.

This leads to the other bodhicitta, the ultimate bodhicitta. This is the great bliss of spiritual liberation—when your entire concern goes beyond self to benefiting all beings. And revealing the great bliss of ultimate bodhicitta depends on experiencing the everyday bliss of relative bodhicitta. This process emphasizes the essence of tantra—working with our mundane human minds and bodies to reveal our enlightened Buddha Nature. For example, the most effective way to discover the selflessness of all phenomena is through your own self. First, you understand you have a self; then you meditate on the emptiness of self; and then you understand the selflessness of self and other and everything. In that way, the self helps you realize selflessness, which is the ultimate wisdom of spiritual liberation. Within our bodies, we have the aforementioned happy hormones, and we increase these through increasing relative bodhicitta. However, these hormones are more than chemical; they are also linked to energy substances within our energy body. We actually have specific energy drops that are antidotes for desire, anger, and ignorance, the three main mental poisons. As you practice Karmamudra, and other practices, these drops wash away emotional imprints of desire, anger, and ignorance so bliss flows freely through your energy body. You use practices within your mundane physical body, like you use mental meditation on the self, to realize and reveal your enlightened energy body, which is the ultimate bodhicitta of spiritual liberation.

Through Karmamudra, you work with the energy concentrated in the lower gate of the body, the genital gate. Through Mahamudra, you work with the energy concentrated in the upper gate of the body, the head gate. So if you aren't interested in Karmamudra, don't worry. You can energetically open the gate of your genitals or the gate of your head. Either way, you get the same result of free-flowing great bliss and its display of altruistic responsiveness and compassionate creativity.

This great bliss of ultimate bodhicitta is different than relative bodhicitta. This great bliss is endless; it is an unending energy resource beyond deterioration. It is free; it is completely free of causes and conditions like self, other, time, and space. It is nondual and all pervasive; it is not separate from self or other or anything. It is beyond imagination; it can only be experienced through meditation. It is beyond description; its nature escapes words. It is the original state. You were born with this bliss. You live with this bliss. You will die with this bliss. You were born as a buddha. You live as a buddha. You will die as a buddha. This great bliss is within you, waiting to be discovered. All you need to do is realize who and what you actually are—a buddha.

With committed and continued practice of Karmamudra, you can discover this great bliss of ultimate bodhicitta. You can realize and reveal your Buddha Nature. Some call Karmamudra liberation without meditation. Normally, many people say they don't have time for meditation, but they always have time for sex. Because when you are in that sexy chemistry and deep desire, even the busy and the lazy will find time for sex. With Karmamudra, you can play with that desire to effortlessly enter into spiritual liberation.

Whatever becomes your practice of choice, you do not ignore your body on the tantric path. It is through your current existence in this human body that you can attain enlightenment. You can be the buddha you already are. You can be of tremendous benefit through your bodhicitta display of the Four Immeasurables—unconditional loving kindness, universal compassion, infinite joy, and unending equanimity. As you nourish yourself into balance, you can nourish our world as well.

DEDICATION

At the end of all Tantric Buddhist practices, it is customary to say a dedication prayer. Generally speaking, this prayer dedicates your practice to be of benefit to all beings. In this lineage, you request that this practice helps you quickly achieve the same enlightened state as Yuthok, and through this may you bring all beings into this state of enlightenment.

Without the dedication prayer, your practice is like a drop of water that falls in the dirt and dries up. With the dedication prayer, your practice is like a drop of water that falls in the ocean and continues to be of benefit evermore.

On that note, thank you for reading this chapter. Regardless of whether you explore this spiritual path, may the commentary on these practices be of great benefit to you and all those you encounter. May you be well and rest easy. May you float through life like the gentle breeze you are.

"*Be flexible and humble.*"

\- Dr. Nida Chenagtsang

Chapter Four – Fire

Recall a time when you were alone in nature. You were sitting or walking. The air was chilled. You were chilled. Then the sun came out. Maybe you were up early and met the dawn. You watched the world come to life. The sky was ablaze with orange and red. Animals appeared, beckoned by the ultimate alarm clock. Maybe you felt the physical warmth and spiritual thrill of meeting the morning's first moment. Or maybe you were out and about on a rainy day, wet and cold, when the clouds parted. Maybe you felt a sunbeam land upon you and bring a smile to your face. Maybe you took off your jacket, feeling renewed and ready for anything. Or maybe you've experienced the magic of not noticing cloud cover until the wind shifts and the world suddenly becomes brighter. Maybe you wondered with laugh, "Who turned up the lights?" Maybe that happens with your mind, too.

Fire lights up our lives. It is the force that drives us forward. With fire running through our being, we are lit. We are excited, assertive, and responsible. We see what needs to be done and we do it. And we're right about it. Fire gives us incisive intelligence, quick learning, and clear thinking. We listen carefully and remember details. We have precise and direct communication. We know what needs to be said and we aren't afraid to say it. No wonder we are so confident in ourselves. And no wonder others are so confident in us. This confidence within and around us makes us magnetic. We can fire up a crowd. We can fire up a movement. We can fire up a romance. Fire knows how to whip up passion, and it always hits its mark.

Similarly, in our physiology, fire makes shit happen, literally. Fire energy is the powerhouse of our digestion. With fire in the belly, we have sun shining on our gut garden, so we can eat a wide range of foods, keep the nutrients we need, and send the waste packing. The fire energy that helps us move our bowels also helps us move with purpose through the world. With fire inside, we feel safe, athletic, and self-assured. Fire also turns on the lights—in our eyes and minds. It supports clear physical vision and clear mental vision. Fire makes the mind quick, shrewd, and analytical. Further, fire gives us a glowing complexion with radiant skin. It's no wonder we're so magnetizing—we literally light up a room. And, of course, fire enlivens the heart. It gives us the courage and strength to fulfill our desires. Fire is the engine of our physical and existential existence.

When fire energy is imbalanced, we go from warm to watch out. We go up in flames. Even if you are not a fire type, you need to pay attention to fire imbalance because we live in a fiery world and fire dominates the bulk of our lives, from adolescence through middle age. With fire imbalance, we are easily irritated and quick to enrage. We embody anger-management issues. Our sporty sense of play heats up to make everything a winner-take-all competition. We become combative and hostile, creating arguments just to win them. We go from responsible to resentful, taking on as much work as possible to prove our point. And what was our point? That I am the best. We become indignant, impatient, and easily disgusted. How could this be happening to me? We become proud and egocentric. Don't you know who I am? Alas, it must be said—narcissism rides on imbalanced fire energy. Just as the earth has a hot, dense center, we become the hot, dense center of our own little world. This elevated ego often comes with an elevated body temperature and inflammation. As the personality becomes stinky, so does the body with bad breath, foul-smelling urine and feces, and profuse and pungent sweating. Our sharp, aggressive emotional reactions are not unlike our acute, sudden physical pains. That healthy glow congeals into oily skin and all-over dampness. And our superpower of hearty and stable digestion gives way to the drama queen of diarrhea with her explosive tendencies. All to say, fire imbalance comes on quick and leaves a mark.

Accordingly, when your fire element is imbalanced, your primary mental toxin is anger. With your mind, body, and energy feeling the heat, you look for someone to blame. And you can always find a target. From parents to partners, from colleagues to strangers, it's not hard to use your incisive intellect to build a case of you-versus-them with every chance you get. You might even pull people in with your charming glow only to shit all over them. Or maybe that's too messy. Maybe you just feel fuck-it about everything. Fuck all of it. Your simmering anger spills out over the whole bloody mess of life. Whether it's an inferno or an ember, that anger is there—isolating you from others, isolating you from yourself, isolating you from all of it, and, ironically, robbing your life of light.

When the poison is anger, what is the medicine? It is detoxing. Rather than putting your shit out onto everyone else, you let that shit out from within. And, of course, we are talking about shit in the broadest sense—all the unnecessary mental, emotional, and physical stuff you've got cooking. Fire energy has a purgative and cleansing nature, which you can use to detox yourself from toxic anger. You can detox through diet and lifestyle. And you can detox through spiritual practice. When you detox, you are balanced. And you feel brighter. From that balance and brightness, you can offer fire's enlivening spirit to be of benefit to us all.

DIET AND LIFESTYLE

Here is the diet-and-lifestyle pith instruction for fire types: Take a seat or a stroll in the shade with some cool water. When your mind chatters, tell your thoughts to the trees until you're bored of your blah blahs. It can be that easy.

Fire types, and those with fire imbalance, thrive with a regular, relaxing lifestyle that includes physical activity. Whatever mental chatter is feeding your flames of discontent, you can move it out of you, but be aware that stress release is the motivation. Otherwise, your release becomes another requirement. Instead of swimming some laps or running a few miles or catching a yoga class or going for a bike ride, you will find a way to win at it. You will learn and lead and train and teach, and then you're back to cooking up stress instead of burning it off. So aim for noncompetitive sports and clear your mind through your body. You do well with seven to eight hours of sleep, and seven to eight hours of work, which can be physical or mental. Even if your work is physical, you may still need exercise in order to release your day. Try not to fill your free time with more work. Find a great book—a nonfiction book that lets you learn in a way unrelated to your work or a novel that lets you mentally wash away your work. Cool and shady places probably feel nice, especially when you're all fired up. You do well with moderate sexual activity, partnered or solo. Sauna sweats are your friend but so are cold plunges as well as cold compresses for pinpointed pain. It would feel good to get to know your breath—watching it will deepen it. But don't beat yourself up if calm abiding meditation doesn't come easily. You don't need to win at meditation. And your analytical mind is well suited for analytical meditation, which we will discuss in a bit.

As part of your regular and relaxing lifestyle, you do well with consistent meals that match your consistent appetite. Maintain a happy gut microbiome with a diverse diet incorporating all of the tastes. In general, fresh and cooling foods work well for fire types. Fresh cool water and fresh fruit juice are great options for you. Green tea and black tea are good when you want caffeine, but take note as to whether caffeine is a medicine or poison for you depending on the amount and time of day. For vegetables, be the bunny and eat the whole garden—leafy greens, carrots, cucumbers, celery, zucchini, squashes, corn, broccoli, cabbage, bell peppers, tomatoes, peas, beets. Create the brightest, freshest salad whenever you can. For fruits, try apples, peaches, pears, lemons, dates, melons, and tropical fruits. You do well with rice, millet, quinoa, lentils, oats, and buckwheat. If you want meat, beef and pork work for you. Oils and dairy can be great for fire—fresh butter, ghee, olive oil, almond oil, coconut oil, milk, yogurt, kefir, fresh cheese, and plant-based dairy alternatives. For spices, turmeric is a friend of fire; it detoxes the liver where anger lives. Saffron is also super for liver detoxification. You can put a tiny bit of saffron in some water, just enough to turn it yellow. It will cool you and calm you down. Mint, parsley, cilantro, coriander, and basil are also great for fire types. Above all, please celebrate your pooping superpower. If you can poop it, you can eat it. Enjoy!

But don't go overboard. Your hearty digestion is not a green light to let non-nutritious food and alcohol become your confused coping mechanism. Every element has their emotional doorway into addiction. For fire types, it tends to be the well-worn victim song of poor me, poor me, pour me another. Yes, things have gone wrong in your life. Yes, people have let you down and hurt you. Yes, you have a lot of responsibilities. Yes, you feel pain and pressure. Sadly, food and alcohol are never going to give you the recognition or even revenge you are seeking. Addiction will just draw you further into your fire, stoking your sadness into anger. And you may know the Buddhist saying about anger—it's like drinking poison and hoping someone else will suffer. You never let anything out by taking more in. The real way to burn off the sadness, disappointment, anger, and even narcissism is through seeing all those flames for what they are—just energy. And there are much better and brighter uses of that energy. And you love to be productive! So, when you're ready, please put down the drink or whatever is holding you back. Honestly, you're too smart to keep going down a dead-end path. Especially because, in your heart of hearts, you know there is a spiritual path that can give you the insight you need to release yourself from anger and reveal yourself as a light unto our world.

SPIRITUAL PRACTICE

Now we will transition into spiritual medicine for fire. Maybe you have never thought of spirituality as something that could detox you. But it can. We will look at Ngöndro practices, pre-empowerment practices, and post-empowerment practices of Guru Yoga/creation stage and completion stage—all with a focus on detoxing and balancing fire. Please note that what follows is a unique commentary on these practices. Of course, there is some instruction within the commentary. However, to practice Ngöndro, Guru Yoga, creation stage, and completion stage, you need a teacher to give you a reading transmission of the root text along with practice instructions. For now, you can explore the potential of these practices from the perspective of detoxing and balancing to consider how the Yuthok Nyingthig could help you be of benefit to yourself and others.

NGÖNDRO

Refuge

You can't win. This is the truth. Do not mistake it for the sad truth because it is the happy truth. This is the truth that sets you free. For a long time, you thought you could win. You have won a lot of things. You're a winner, generally speaking. And when you don't win, you know that closed doors mean open windows and rejection is protection and all that don't stop believing blah blah blah. But, blessedly, at some point, you won't win. The work world wears on you. The health scare scares you. The lover leaves you. The kid confounds you. The erection escapes you. Whatever it is, it will happen. You can try your tactics of winning some other way or rebelling some shadowy way, but you will still end up with yourself and your thoughts and your pain and your anger. And it hurts. But this good—because now your life can actually begin. You can step out of the hamster wheel, you can see through the dream, you can release the conditioning, and you can stop suffering. You can stop wasting your time taking refuge in winning things that don't actually bring you lasting happiness. Instead, you can take refuge in your spiritual path, and you can get to work, for real.

For you, dear fiery one, this first step might be the biggest step. Because you need to admit that you can't do this alone. You need help. You need help from a teacher. You need help from the teachings. You even, ugh, need help from your peers, and some of those peers are, ugh, already further along on the path. Make no mistake; this first step of taking refuge in the Buddha, Dharma, and Sangha can be a big slice of humble pie. But you have great digestion! Once you see the truth, you are so smart and so sharp that your mind can process the situation. You can happily take the slice of humble pie and devour the entire delicious menu.

This is when the relief sets in. It feels so good to finally admit that you need help—and to find this help. There is a teacher. There are teachings. There is community. In this world of marketing and made-up masters, you have stumbled upon an actual reliable source of refuge in the Buddha, Dharma, and Sangha. Go ahead and do the research, kick the tires, and see how the whole thing feels. Then settle in and enjoy the ride. Find the ease in the medicine and the sweetness in a taste of faith. Even better, thanks to tantra, you don't need to abandon your job or your car or your clothes or your 401k or your kid's college-savings plan. You can still do all your stuff, but your relationship to it all changes. It will no longer be your source of confused refuge because it has never worked and it never will. So stop wasting time and start waking up.

Bodhicitta

When fire types do something, you want to do it right. So here you go. If you want to take flight on this path, you need two wings—wisdom and compassion, also known as emptiness and bodhicitta. This is the essence of the Buddhadharma. You need to understand, really understand, that everything's nature is emptiness. The entire material dimension—you, me, everything—is waves of interconnected energy that are constantly transforming. Nothing is solid, fixed, or real in the dualistic way you are seeing it now. As you understand this, you start to wake up. You start to see glimpses that every problem you have is empty because you are empty and so are all the people and things involved in your problems. And this is true for everyone. You start to see the extraordinary and overlapping messes we are all making by not understanding emptiness. You won't quite know how to act on this awareness because understanding emptiness is not the same as realizing emptiness and there is a lot of conditioning to burn through. But one big thing will happen—your heart will break. And this is the dawn of bodhicitta. You will want to do whatever you can to truly put an end to the suffering brought on by the ignorance of dualism. You will want to get enlightened for the benefit of all beings. And, through this wish, you will start to develop both of your wings.

Otherwise, you are talking about spirituality and philosophy or doing yoga and meditation or taking plant medicines and dancing in trances or whatever you are doing to feel a little relief for yourself, but even if you get a visceral hit of emptiness here and there, you are barely flapping one wing. And that is fine. But you will not take flight. That only happens when your heart breaks open and you want to practice spirituality to be of benefit to every single sentient being without exception. Every human. Every animal. Every bug. Every being. In fact, you will happily stay in the mess with pain and problems while watching everyone else wake up and fly off because you are committed to being here for the awakening of every single being. When you are willing to be left behind because you will leave no one behind, then we are talking about the Buddhadharma. Then you have two wings. You don't need to call yourself a Buddhist. That is not the point. The point is these two wings—wisdom and compassion, emptiness and bodhicitta.

So if you want to do this for real, you begin each practice by reminding yourself of your altruistic motivation of bodhicitta. And you attempt to embody the Six Perfections of generosity, morality, effort, patience, meditation, and wisdom. You stay on the ground and you practice unfurling your two baby-chicky wings. Do this and you will fly soon enough.

The Four Immeasurables

It is not easy to grow these two wings in the belly of individualism. This is why you have the booster shot of the Four Immeasurables. The Four Immeasurables prayer in the Yuthok Nyingthig is a series of sentences that are spoken and contemplated:

May all beings have happiness and the causes of happiness.
May all beings be free from suffering and the causes of suffering.
May all beings never be separated from the supreme joy
that is beyond all suffering.
May all beings abide in equanimity, free from attachment,
aversion, and sorrow.

You know the Four Immeasurables prayer is working when you start to forget your own problems. This is because you are seriously contemplating the situations of others. We always think that our lives are full of problems, and we are trained these days to blah blah about our problems. And you do have problems. And it is important to discuss some problems. But if we have the privilege to contemplate the Four Immeasurables, if we have the privilege to even hear of the Four Immeasurables, then our problems, as serious as they are, are not as serious as the majority of humanity's problems, let alone all sentient beings. Countless human beings do not have shelter or food. They are starving and sick. They are suffering through poverty and war. If we truly compare our lives with billions of other humans, we will get some perspective on our problems and we will generate genuine empathy for others. I often tell people to practice the Four Immeasurables until you lose tears. If you don't cry at first, it's okay. But there will come a time for tears. Because if you really let yourself think about what is happening to other human beings, you will feel love and compassion for them. You will want to take advantage of your precious human rebirth to do something meaningful and worthwhile that is of benefit to those human beings. You will grow feathers on your fledgling wings.

Of course, the Four Immeasurables prayer says "all beings," so you can extend this love and compassion to all animals and insects and unseen beings. But you know what is an even more nutritious supplement for fire types? To contemplate the Four Immeasurables for those who have done you wrong. Remember the saying about anger—it is like swallowing poison and hoping someone else will suffer. So what could be better medicine than sending well wishes to those who piss you off? It's like taking a love laxative so you can poop out all your anger. How detoxifying!

You don't need to start with this. It is an advanced practice. However, when you are ready, give it a try. Bring to mind the ex, the boss, the frenemy, the rude guy in line and say:

> *May you have happiness and the causes of happiness.*
> *May you be free from suffering and the causes of suffering.*
> *May you never be separated from the supreme joy*
> *that is beyond all suffering.*
> *May you abide in equanimity, free from attachment,*
> *aversion, and sorrow.*

Because what does it cost you to make these wishes? The only thing you have to lose is toxic anger and its sneaky sidekick pride. What you have to gain is the freedom of two big fluffy wings.

Prostrations

In their physicality, prostrations are some of the best medicine available for fire types. Fire types tend to have socially desirable bodies—athletic and well proportioned with erect posture. So you might have been trained by societal approval to focus on your body. Maybe you know you look good and use that to your advantage. Maybe you feel fast and strong and a little superior because of it. Maybe you succeed in sports and enjoy that stature. Maybe you feel pressure to maintain your hot body. Maybe you spend precious energy preening and primping. Maybe you want to surround your beautiful body in luxury. Maybe you spend a lot of time thinking about your body, caring for your body, showing off your body, worrying about your body, using your body, even abusing your body, all in the name of having a so-called good body and all that goes with that. All to say, for most fire types, your body plays a starring role in your stories of I and self.

Now, through the genius of tantra, you get to use you to undo you. A lot of fire types initially feel great about doing prostrations. Not for the devotional aspect but for the athletic aspect. You feel good doing prostrations. You look good doing prostrations. You like the challenge of prostrations. Initially, prostrations seem like contemporary yoga where you work your abs, arms, and butt while doing supposed spiritual practice—score!

And then prostrations get boring. And then prostrations get painful. And then prostrations seem endless. And then prostrations seem pointless. And then the cracks in your devotion show.

Maybe you get frustrated wasting time doing athletic activity that isn't recharging in the way you want athletic activity to be. Maybe you question bowing before anything. Maybe you think this practice is antiquated. Maybe you are annoyed with the teacher. Maybe you feel angry. Maybe you feel betrayed because this practice was supposed to detox your anger. Maybe you wonder what the eff you're doing.

This is the moment to call on that fire discipline and stay with the medicine. This process is like lancing a boil. It might not be pretty, but it works. And you will know it is working when you realize you can't do this the way you've done everything else. You have to put your trust in the teacher. You have to put your trust in the teachings. You have to put your trust in all the others who have gone through this. You have to let the prostrations do you.

Then, the you that is invested in workouts and beauty and praise and all such stories of I and self, that you fades away. You realize that nothing—no compliments received, no confidence displayed, no challenge met—feels better than being a body of sublime offering to the Buddha, Dharma, and Sangha. And with that, you truly and deeply and joyfully say:

From whose kindness great bliss itself instantly arises within us,
the guru with jewel-like form, holder of the vajra,
I prostrate at your feet.

Mandala

I have a student who works in fashion design. When she started to practice Buddhism, she went to a variety of centers and temples. Once, as she entered a monastery, she suddenly became self-conscious about her Gucci bag. Was it wrong to have a Gucci bag in a monastery? Was it wrong to have a Gucci bag and be Buddhist? And it wasn't just this one Gucci bag that troubled her. She had plenty of beautiful bags and clothes and shoes, not to mention her cool apartment. She wondered if her things fit within Buddhism. She wondered if she fit within Buddhism. Then she encountered tantra and the Yuthok Nyingthig and Mandala offering practice. She learned that she didn't need to give up her bags, clothes, shoes, and apartment, but, with the wisdom of non-attachment, she could change her relationship to them. She learned that she could own things without things owning her. So she kept her Gucci bag and the rest, holding them lightly and celebrating them as an offering.

Fire types tend to be successful in the ways of the world. With your disciplined and hardworking nature, chances are you have had material success and have some nice stuff to show for it. Good for you. Enjoy your stuff. Enjoy your life. And celebrate it all as a glorious visualized offering in Mandala practice. This can be a win-win—you get to keep your beloved stuff and you get to offer it to the guru. Use your sharp mind to create a vivid visualization of all your favorite things. Offer it completely to your teachers and gurus with no attachment. Then visualize its complete dissolution. Over and over, you create, offer, dissolve. Slowly slowly, you will understand the lesson learned by the student with her Gucci bag—you can own things without things owning you. This medicine of non-attachment will help you feel more relaxed about your things. Your things will no longer demand that you maintain a wall of perfectionism and stress around them. The spill on your carpet? It's all good. The ding in your car? It's all good. You can have a spacious sense of ease with all of your beautiful things. You understand things as an offering. And offerings come. And offerings go. All of this might expand your mind to see your life as a beautiful offering that also does not demand a wall of perfectionism and stress around it. Maybe it's possible to own your life without your life owning you?

Circumambulation

With your fiery go-getter spirit, you can enjoy circumambulation as a melding of Mandala, prostrations, and the Four Immeasurables. First, feel free to do one long circumambulation by going for your usual run or hike or swim or walk or ride, now with Medicine Buddha visualized over your right shoulder while you say his mantra, audibly or silently—TADYATA OM BEKADZE BEKADZE MAHA BEKADZE RADZA SAMUDGATE SOHA. In so doing, the world around you becomes an offering to Medicine Buddha, just like Mandala. And, of course, your body that is circumambulating becomes its own offering, just like prostrations. Now you are no longer simply working out. Now you are generating vast merit and blessings for you and all you encounter. More and more, anytime you do anything, you can feel the presence of Medicine Buddha as well as the mantra flowing through your mind. In this way, your entire life starts to feel like an offering. You practice tantra—being the continuation of the wave of awakening in the world. Of course, the last step is to not limit this experience to you. To truly be the wave of tantra, you include all beings in your circumambulations and your daily comings and goings with Medicine Buddha by your side. You can think about those you love and let them join you in these blessings. And, of course, you can think about those you don't love and don't like and don't want to think about and let them join you in these blessings. Don't forget to think about those who make you angry, dear fiery one. Truth be told, you think about them anyway. However, now instead of simmering about them, you surround them with a spacious state of mind and a healing mantra. In this way, all of these people are helping you become a messenger of Medicine Buddha. Notice how this affects your thoughts, your speech, and your actions as you make your way in the world.

Vajrasattva

Vajrasattva was made for detoxing, literally. He is the buddha of purification. If there was ever a practice to clear out your shit, it is Vajrasattva. Again, in this practice, Vajrasattva rests above your head. He embodies nonjudgmental compassion, and his blessings flow through your body as healing nectar. Traditionally, Vajrasattva is white, as is the nectar, but go with whatever color feels cleansing for you. In that vein, you can see and feel the nectar as liquid or light—whatever works for you. If you would rather see Vajrasattva as a ball of light, again go with whatever works for you. The point is that you have a reservoir of healing energy in your crown chakra, and, with the help of Vajrasattva, you can tap into that healing energy and spread it throughout your body. As you visualize the nectar flowing through you, you say Vajrasattva's mantra, and whatever you want to release leaves your body as visualized smoke or sludge or whatever appears to your mind. It all exits through your orifices and pores. Let the nectar flow in and let the shit flow out.

Now let's talk more specifically about the shit, shall we. We have talked about fire's main toxin of anger, but the fire of anger has a lot of flames. Clearly, anger can display as aggressive, hostile, and combative behavior. And woe is the being receiving that fiery rage. But anger can also display as passive-aggressive behavior and too-cool-for-school detachment. And woe is the being facing fire's cold shoulder. Then there is fire's charm offensive—the manipulation and seduction to get what we want. Who can resist the sunshine of fire's attention? But then there is the casting out should that charm offensive fail. And who can survive the darkness of fire's dismissal? Of course, when fire energy is imbalanced, what we do to others in anger doesn't hold a candle to what we do to ourselves. Inner anger and its flames of perfectionism, self-hate, mental and even physical torture can be the stuff of hell realms. We rule ourselves with an iron fist, and it hurts us and then we hurt others.

Now is the time to cool it, dear fiery one. In your wisdom of emptiness, you know that angry flames are only energy—habitual patterns of mental movement. With Vajrasattva, you don't need to think through where the patterns came from or why the patterns stick around or even how the patterns harm self and other. You simply receive nonjudgmental compassion in the form of healing nectar and let it do its thing. Relax and receive. That's it. Give it time. There is a reason this practice is included in Ngöndro. Many, many, many practitioners have healed from the poison of anger by relaxing and allowing Vajrasattva to wash it all away.

Kusali Body Offering

Then you have an offering party. Fire types may present as all business, but fire energy also likes a party. During Chöd, your visualized consciousness exits your body and becomes a sexy, fiery-red wisdom deity. And if anyone knows how to party, it's her. She is hosting a feast for the ages. Everyone is welcome—the ones you love, the ones you shun, the ones you hate, the ones you venerate. A good party needs a good mix of energies, so you don't turn anyone away. Let that sexy, fiery-red wisdom deity invite all the guests to enjoy the nectar of your body. Whatever they want, the nectar is it.

You have worked hard at Ngöndro. You have done all the things. Now you get to release your constructs and your categories and get wild. And why not? You're practicing being a buddha and bringing every being exactly what they need. Did you think compassionate action was all work and no play? Hell no! That sexy, fiery-red wisdom deity is always smiling and laughing while she wears a barely there dress and charms the pants off her guests. And you know a thing or two about charming people, don't you, dear fiery one? But the difference between your mundane expression and your wisdom expression is that wisdom is never seducing. Wisdom does not need anything from the guests; she gets off on universal compassion. She is here for the dance party of nondualism—no giver, no receiver, no gift. So tear up the memo of poor-me stories, tear up the ledger of who-owes-you-what, tear up the playbook of you-versus-them. For a moment, let it all go up in flames and feel what is. Ah.

PRE-EMPOWERMENT PRACTICE

Analytical Meditation

Have you ever tried to meditate and then thought you can't meditate because you can't stop thinking? Well, you're in luck. Because now you can do thinking meditation! This is actually a thing. And it is a perfect thing for fire types with your critical thinking skills. The bonus is you will build up those fluffy wings of wisdom and compassion. The double bonus is you will learn that thinking isn't a problem after all—during meditation or otherwise. You only think that thinking is a problem if you haven't learned how to think in a way that frees you. So now, dear fiery one, let's leverage your superpower of sharp thinking to free yourself and others.

To do so, you can experiment with two analytical meditation methods. The first will increase your understanding of interdependence.

The second will increase your understanding of emptiness. Remember that understanding interdependence and emptiness reveals more of your inherent wisdom, the feminine principle, which will then birth more compassion, the masculine principle.

For the interdependence meditation, you are going to use your incisive intelligence to pull apart a situation into some of its countless component pieces. To address imbalanced fire's main toxin of anger, you can contemplate a situation where you are angry with someone. Let's be honest, you are probably stewing over this situation already. So make it a detox stew. To that end, dedicate a regular time for your analytical meditation. Find a position that is comfortable—sitting or lying down or walking if the situation has you too heated to be still. Set a timer for five or ten minutes; keep it short to start. Then, in a methodical manner, think about the causes and conditions that have contributed to this situation where you are angry with someone.

Start by heating up the spices. Look at the immediate issues, such as what you said and did and what they said and did. Then add the soffritto for a base. Look at why you said and did those things. This can include your emotions about the situation as well as other interactions you had around that time and also things like your stress, sleeping, eating, digestion, and exercise. Then add the meat that makes up most of your stews. Look at your personality and your elemental typology and your thought, speech, and behavior patterns and how it all flavors your interactions with others, including this situation. Then add the broth it all cooks in. Look at how your personality and patterns were formed; consider your culture, education, and family history. Stir this up as much as you would like. Then add the particular veggies for this stew. Look at the other(s) involved in the situation. Granted, you probably don't know their details—from the prosaic of their personal pooping patterns to the horrific of their grandparents' historical traumas—but you are a human and you know the things that humans go through. So you can find all the fixings to complete the meal.

And here is the final and essential instruction. You have to keep the stove on simmer. Do not let your mind rest for a moment during this meditation. Not one moment!

Repeat this process with this same situation for days, weeks, months until you feel complete. You will know you are complete when: 1) you see the entire spread, the profound complexity of the causes and conditions at play, such that it is impossible to solidify the situation into simply you-versus-them, and 2) you feel so satiated by this situation that if a whiff of it arises, your mind is like an old dog that doesn't even lift its head to acknowledge the smell.

Left to its standard fare of dualistic ignorance, your mind would stew over this anger story again and again to solidify you-versus-them. In fact, it is through such simplified stories of anger or desire that we all create concepts of self and other as well as us and them. We do this constantly and reflexively; it is the go-to menu of mind. With this interdependence meditation, you can liberate yourself from leftover habitual dualism. Instead, you will feast on the fresh perspective of interdependence with its complex notes and surprising tastes. With this wisdom revealed, you will feel great compassion for all of us who are still eating the scraps of what came before.

The emptiness meditation naturally follows the fullness of the interdependence meditation. As thoughts arise, simply look at them. Look at the nature of thoughts. With your keen fire vision, I'll bet you no longer see thoughts as a problem because you see right through them.

In fact, if you want to explore more, notice what happens when you don't hold on to a thought. Usually, we invite a thought to stay, offer it a seat and a cup of tea, and then ask it to bring its whole family of thoughts to dinner so we can sit around the table for hours and tell a big story. But if you don't extend the thought an invitation to stay, it will walk away. In meditation terminology, we say that thoughts self-liberate.

You know what else self-liberates? The self. Because the self is only continuous stories made of continuous thoughts. The self is an enormous Italian dinner of thoughts with an aperitivo of family history, antipasto of childhood curiosity, primo of teenage drama, secondo of adult responsibility, dolce of bittersweet elderhood, and a digestivo to wash it all down. So, please remember, you are actively cooking up this self of stories. You can make it easy to digest.

Three-Part Purification Breathing

Think about what you are angry about all the time. What is your top toxic anger? What is your daily dammit? Now imagine your anger as an animal. Are you a viper preparing to strike? Are you a shark preparing to bite? Are you a cat preparing to scratch? Choose an animal to represent this anger. Choose whatever you would like.

Then prepare to release that animal from your being and with it all of your anger. You can do this through a three-part breathing exercise. Take a smooth inhale, gently retain the breath for a moment, and on the exhale visualize a zillion of your anger animals leaving the body through all of your orifices and pores. Vamos, vipers. Sayonara, sharks. Catch ya later, cats. Smooth inhale, gentle retention, exhale the animals. If you want a sound to go with it, silently say "OM" on the inhale, "AH" on the retention, and "HUNG" on the exhale. If you want a color to go with it, visualize white light entering you on the inhale, red light spreading through you on the retention, and blue light leaving you with the animals on the exhale. Or choose other soothing sounds and colors. Or use the sounds and colors but not the animal visualization. Do it whenever you want or as a formal practice for a few minutes each day. Don't overthink it.

Mantra Healing

As mentioned, mantra, or mind protection, is a form of self-therapy. To detox with mantra, shout it from the rooftops. Actually, if you can, go somewhere private—a nature spot or your home or your car—and let 'er rip. Instead of yelling all the habitual things you want to yell, yell the mantra with full force. It will discharge energy without getting you into trouble. A simple and powerful mantra is OM AH HUNG, which was suggested for the breathing exercise above. You can start there and see how it goes.

POST-EMPOWERMENT PRACTICE – CREATION STAGE

Inner Guru Yoga

Inner Guru Yoga presents another opportunity to use your sharp thinking for self-liberation, but this time in a more artistic manner. Fire types tend to have detail-oriented minds capable of vivid visualizations and insightful analysis. As compared to Outer Guru Yoga, Inner Guru Yoga gives your mind more to play with in terms of activity and symbolism. And, as your mind explores the visualization, your body and energy may have illuminating experiences of their own. You may uncover more clarity regarding the specifics of spiritual enlightenment. In fact, this practice is officially known as the source of the fulfillment of all wishes—whatever you want, whatever you need, whatever you desire, it all comes to you through Inner Guru Yoga because you have had it within you all along.

Before describing the practice, here is a special note for fire types. When you meditate, please do not stress. While fire types tend to be capable of vivid visualizations and insightful analysis, you also tend to get stuck in perfectionism. In meditation, if you worry about whether you are sitting correctly or not, breathing correctly or not, chanting correctly or not, imagining correctly or not, then it is hard to relax and actually meditate. In the meditation instructions, Yuthok reassures you not to worry if the directions say one thing and your mind does another—for example, you are supposed to see red and you see blue, you are supposed to feel something in your throat and you sense it outside your body. Try to follow the instructions but trust that whatever you are doing is fine. Relax and allow your practice, and life, to sort itself out.

Inner Guru Yoga can be done as a seven-day retreat and a daily practice. Either way, each time you begin a session, sit in a comfortable position and recite Refuge, Bodhicitta, and the Four Immeasurables. That will establish an altruistic motivation and good foundation for your practice.

Then transform yourself into light-filled Medicine Buddha—or whatever buddha or deity you choose. Remember, Yuthok gives you the freedom to regenerate in a way that resonates for you. Medicine Buddha is blue, which is a healing and calming color that can chill out fire types. He is sitting in lotus position, though you need not be. In his right hand, he holds an arura plant, which cures all diseases. In his left hand, he holds a bowl containing healing nectar. As Medicine Buddha, you can wear a fancy robe or a simple robe, jewels or no jewels. You choose your display because you are displaying the truth of the buddha you are. The most important thing is to see yourself, and sense yourself, as a completely empty body of light.

Then you visualize a channel of light, the circumference of a bamboo tube, running vertically through the center of your buddha body, from your crown point to your pelvic floor. It is white on the outside and red on the inside and crystal clear. Just as you truly are a buddha, you also truly have this central channel within your energy body. You are simply bringing attention to it now.

Then red light emanates from your heart center and travels down your central channel and out your anus. Once the light leaves your body, it expands into a flat red disc, upon which you are seated. You can imagine this solar disc to be as big as your meditation space, your home, the country, the world, or the universe.

Then another light emanates from your heart center and travels down your central channel and out your urethra. Once the light leaves your body, it becomes two crossed vajras. When the vajras hit the solar disc, they melt and expand up and around you, creating a spherical tent of protection. You can make this vajra tent as large as you would like. Try to see it and sense it all around you. Inside this tent, you are completely protected. If you believe in bad spirits or harmful energies or negative thoughts, you are totally safe from these things now. You can relax and focus on your meditation.

To increase your safety and security and blessings and power, you then invite all of your buddhas, gurus, and teachers into the vajra tent. Buddhas of compassion, wisdom, power, purification, they are all here. Male and female buddhas, buddhas in union, peaceful buddhas and wrathful buddhas, they are all here. All of your gurus and teachers, they are all here. What do you naturally do when all of your spiritual supporters show up? Out of gratitude, you again say Refuge and Bodhicitta. Upon hearing your prayers and aspirations, all the buddhas, gurus, and teachers dissolve into you, like snowflakes melting in the sun. Feel their light bodies melting into your light body.

Having prepared yourself and the space, you now enter the heart of the practice. Of course, there are more detailed steps to be given when you receive the official transmission and instructions. For now, it is enough to know that through Inner Guru Yoga you explore the true nature of your five major chakras—the energy centers in your head, throat, heart, navel, and genital area.

As you have physically incarnated in human form this lifetime, your energy body has as well. Your energy body is full of channels, and these channels intersect in chakras, like roads intersecting in traffic circles. Here in your human expression, the channels and chakras have knots, which makes it difficult for your energy to flow smoothly. To be more specific, this blocked energy creates internal poisons—ignorance, desire, anger, pride, and jealousy. And, because mind, body, and energy are all connected, these toxins are then displayed in your thoughts, speech, and actions as well as your health. As discussed, there are a lot of medicines to treat these poisons. One medicinal approach is to detoxify these toxins by releasing the knots. As the knots clear, and energy flows smoothly, your energy body relaxes into its original state as an awakened buddha and your thoughts, speech, and actions follow suit. This can sound a little woo-woo, but think of it like this: How do you feel when you are constipated? Angry, cranky, stuck. How do you feel when you have a super duper poop? Light, joyful, playful. So when your pooping pipes are blocked, you are a sad expression of you; and when your pooping pipes are open, you are a happy expression of you. It's like that on a massive scale. So the prescription here is to clear the knots. And the detox medicine to clear the knots is light.

To that end, this practice is a meditation of visualizing three-dimensional buddhas of bright light in each chakra. You do not say a mantra. You just focus on the light. You visualize a peaceful buddha—lotus posture, simple robe, hands at the navel holding a bowl, topknot of hair, gaze resting down. But if you want to see fancy buddhas wearing jewels or wrathful buddhas or joyful buddhas in union, go for it. As you visualize these buddhas of bright light, your five main toxins in these five main chakras transform into their true nature of five wisdoms.

You start with the heart chakra, which typically has the most knots. Maybe you can feel this? Like your tender heart is under lock and key in this hamster wheel? To help clear all these knots, your heart chakra detoxes with nine buddhas. You visualize an eight-petaled lotus in your heart with a bright blue Medicine Buddha in the center of the lotus and eight other bright blue Medicine Buddhas on the petals surrounding and facing him. The blue light of the buddhas detoxes your heart chakra and transforms anger into clarity—like you do in thinking meditation. Rather than seeing solid targets for your anger, you see the interdependence and emptiness of all phenomena. But don't get too intellectual with Inner Guru Yoga. Quietly let your mind wander all around the three-dimensional Medicine Buddhas. Look at their lotus sitting position, their robes, their bowls, their topknots, their eyes. When your mind wants to rest, focus on one spot on one buddha, like the heart center. As you do this, bright blue light radiates from the Medicine Buddhas to the entire universe. This light has two actions. It offers light to all the buddhas of all times and it purifies the anger of all beings. You relax and meditate on the blue Medicine Buddhas and radiate blue light.

Then you move to the head chakra. This is between your eyebrows. There you visualize a bright white buddha sitting on top of a lotus and white light filling your skull. The white light detoxes your head chakra and transforms ignorance into spaciousness. Rather than shutting out life and hiding from truths you know, you can be with anything and everything in a calm and spacious manner. But, again, no need to get too intellectual. Quietly let your mind wander all around the three-dimensional white buddha. Look at his lotus sitting position, robe, bowl, topknot, eyes. When your mind wants to rest, focus on one spot on the buddha. As you do this, bright white light radiates from the buddha to the entire universe. This light has two actions. It offers light to all the buddhas of all times and it purifies the ignorance of all beings. You relax and meditate on the white buddha and radiate white light.

Then you move to the throat chakra. This is in the center of your throat. There you visualize a bright red buddha sitting on top of a lotus and red light filling your neck. The red light detoxes your throat chakra and transforms desire into awareness. Rather than acquiring things and seducing people out of a need for approval or admiration or anything, you are aware of the beauty of all things and all beings without needing to make them yours. But, again, no need to get too intellectual. Quietly let your mind wander all around the three-dimensional red buddha. Look at his lotus sitting position, robe, bowl, topknot, eyes. When your mind wants to rest, focus on one spot on the buddha. As you do this, bright red light radiates from the buddha to the entire universe. This light has two actions. It offers light to all the buddhas of all times and it purifies the desire of all beings. You relax and meditate on the red buddha and radiate red light.

Then you move to the navel chakra. This is behind the navel in the center of your abdomen. There you visualize a bright yellow buddha sitting on top of a lotus and yellow light filling your abdomen. The yellow light detoxes your navel chakra and transforms pride into equanimity. Rather than always scheming to be the best, you rest in knowing all is well as it is. But, again, no need to get too intellectual. Quietly let your mind wander all around the three-dimensional yellow buddha. Look at his lotus sitting position, robe, bowl, topknot, eyes. When your mind wants to rest, focus on one spot on the buddha. As you do this, bright yellow light radiates from the buddha to the entire universe. This light has two actions. It offers light to all the buddhas of all times and it purifies the pride of all beings. You relax and meditate on the yellow buddha and radiate yellow light.

Then you move to the base chakra. This is in your genitals. There you visualize a bright green buddha on top of a lotus and green light filling your pelvis. However, instead of a peaceful buddha, here you can visualize an active, wrathful buddha, dancing and surrounded by flames. The green light detoxes your base chakra and transforms jealousy into awakened activity. Rather than distracting yourself with mundane self-other stories of lack, you focus on benefiting beings. This wrathful buddha transcends time and space and has a bit of an edge, so you know exactly what to do and when to do it in order to wake up self and other. But, again, no need to get too intellectual. Quietly let your mind wander all around the three-dimensional green buddha. Look at his dancing posture, wild clothes, flying hair, penetrating eyes. When your mind wants to rest, focus on one spot on the buddha. As you do this, bright green light radiates from the buddha to the entire universe. This light has two actions. It offers light to all the buddhas of all times and it purifies the jealousy of all beings. You relax and meditate on the green buddha and radiate green light.

Once you feel complete, you revisit each chakra and dissolve each of the buddhas into light and then into space. And then you, as Medicine Buddha, dissolve into space.

Inner Guru Yoga also includes a completion stage practice. You visualize a very bright white light in your head. Focus on it. Stay with it. Once this light is established, you visualize red light in your throat, blue light in your heart, yellow light in your navel, green light in your base. Or if you see all white lights, that is fine. Without distraction, sleepiness, or too many thoughts, let bright light fill your entire body. In this state of clarity, perhaps even pleasure, keep your mind loose and free from grasping. If thoughts arise, let them arise. If thoughts do not arise, let them not arise. Do not grasp anything. Leave your mind as it is, like a stone on the side of a road. There is no meditation and no meditator. Then dissolve it all into space. Rest.

It is interesting how Outer Guru Yoga and Inner Guru Yoga are connected. With Outer Guru Yoga, you look into a mirror and see your guru. With Inner Guru Yoga, your guru reflects the mirror back at you and you see the guru within yourself. You turn on the lights in your chakras to see what you are. You no longer need to be confused and see yourself as consumed by ignorance, desire, anger, pride, and jealousy. You self-empower to see you have the body, speech, mind, qualities, and activities of all the buddhas. You see the truth.

Whatever you focus on, you will become. When your mind is focused on the five wisdoms of spaciousness, awareness, clarity, equanimity, and awakened activity, there is no room for your afflictive emotions. This meditation directly detoxes your toxins. You can even use it outside of formal practice. When you are spaced out, see the white buddha in your head and feel spaciousness. When you are desirous, see the red buddha in your throat and feel awareness. When you are angry, see the blue buddha in your heart and feel clarity. When you are prideful, see yellow buddha in your navel and feel equanimity. When you are jealous, see the green buddha in your genitals and feel awakened activity. Inner Guru Yoga is a more artistic version of thinking meditation. When you see the light, you see the light. When you feel the light, you feel the light. The light is the moment-by-moment medicine of detoxification. When the buddhas are in your chakras, there are no poisons. That's it. You're free.

POST-EMPOWERMENT PRACTICE – COMPLETION STAGE

Tummo Yoga

In completion stage, you are invited to take detoxing up a notch. Instead of using light as your medicine, you use fire. Tummo means wild and wrathful lady—and this lady is all fire, all the time. She brings the heat, and she brings the bliss.

In the Yuthok Nyingthig, there are three Tummo Yoga practices—mind (meditation), speech (breathing), and body (physical exercises). Depending on what medicine you need, you might only meditate on the visualization or your might add breathing and physical exercises. We will discuss Tummo Yoga in the next chapter as well because Tummo Yoga can be used medicinally for both fire and earth/water types. Really, Tummo Yoga can be medicine for everyone; it is the foundation of

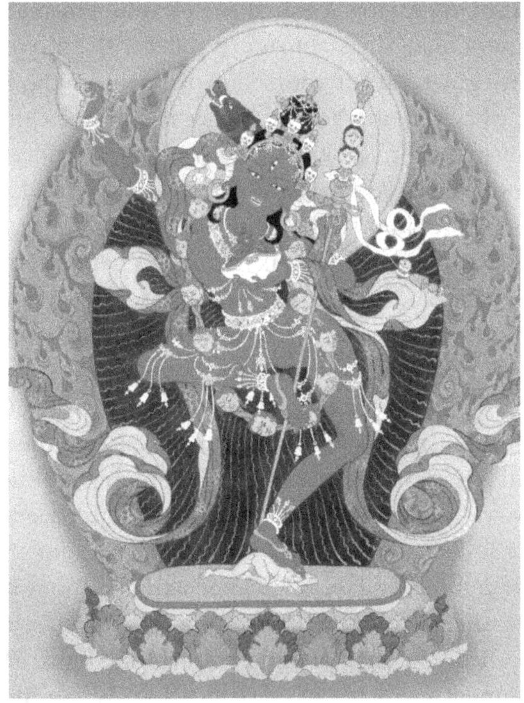

Vajra Yogini

completion stage practice. For fire types, and those with fire imbalance, Tummo Yoga can be homeopathic. Heat cures heat. Also, in general, practices that involve generating as a red-colored being can balance fire energy. However, depending on your fire imbalance, it might be best to only practice Tummo Yoga meditation and maybe some breathing but not the physical exercises because they could create too much heat and increase inflammation. A teacher would be able to help you determine the appropriate approach. Thus, it bears repeating that to practice Tummo Yoga you need transmission and instruction from a qualified teacher within an established lineage. These days, there is a lot of interest in tummo-like practices within popular spirituality and wellness. For the sake of your mind, body, and energy, as well as for the sake of all beings, please be a discerning seeker. On that note, we will only briefly discuss the Tummo Yoga technique here and instead focus more on the fruition.

Tummo Yoga is an alchemical process. Through fire, you transform toxins into bliss. Tummo fire is located four finger-widths below your navel within your central channel. All fires need air and fuel, so you fuel tummo fire with breath and toxins. Similar to Vajrasattva, this is a detox practice. Except now, instead of gentle Vajrasattva washing away your stuff, you generate as a wrathful, fiery-red female deity who is tired of your self-centered bullshit. You know the wise part of you that is ready to kick your own ass? Yes, her. She has been watching you do damage to self and other from the get-go, and she is over it. She is wearing everything you fear as jewelry and laughing about it. She does not play. So please bring your toxins to the fire and let them burn into bliss.

As with all fire, the nature of tummo fire is heat. And you will feel physical heat during this practice. But this is a different heat than you experience when you have imbalanced fire energy or you are ill with a fever. Tummo fire is wisdom heat. It does not disturb you. In fact, it brings you great joy. It does this by heating up a white energy drop at the top of your central channel in your crown point. The nature of this energy drop is bliss. Chances are you are not experiencing bliss at this moment. But that does not mean you do not have bliss. Your body is actually made of blissful energy, but this energy is blocked by the knots of your toxic emotions. When you have an orgasm, it is a big enough bang of bliss to burst through the knots, but then the habitual toxins return. You know how it goes with patterns; they form well-worn grooves. Without those toxins, you could feel a subtle, pleasurable bliss and aliveness all the time. In Inner Guru Yoga, you use light as medicine to clear the knots. In Tummo Yoga, you use fire in this same medicinal way—by creating a blaze of heat and bliss in your central channel and then expanding your central channel throughout your body, and beyond, to clear the knots, detox the toxins, and deliver you into your natural state of all-pervasive bliss.

Through this process, you can meet your body anew. You realize that your brain is made of orgasm, but it is frozen right now. It is frozen and stuck, like the rest of you, which is also made of orgasm. That's what life is—orgasm. You were born with bliss; you live with bliss; you die with bliss. This whole thing could be ongoing orgasm. Now you are interested! But the point of Tummo Yoga is not orgasm in the way you are probably thinking about orgasm. The orgasm talk sparks your interest because you have been conditioned in the hamster wheel where mundane sex sells. But there is wisdom in your confusion. Deep down, you know you are made of bliss; this is why you run around chasing after others who might give you orgasms. Now the wild and wrathful lady is here to show you the truth of your orgasm and yourself—and this truth is Buddha Nature.

When you have an orgasm, the blissful energy is strong enough to momentarily stop your stories of self-creation—stories rooted in ignorance, desire, anger, jealousy, and pride. This is a glimpse of the presence and joy possible when you wake up for real. In addition to body protection and continuation, tantra also means liberation through expansion. When you expand your central channel and all your knots are released and your body is full of bliss, what is coursing through your body? It is bodhicitta! Pure bodhicitta, like a blissful nectar, flowing throughout your body, even beyond your body, as your sense of self expands to the far reaches of the universe. You lose notions of inside and outside. You lose notions of self and other. You lose notions of subject and object. You lose notions of past and present and future. Everything is bliss. Whatever you see is bliss. Whatever you hear is bliss. Whatever you smell is bliss. Whatever you taste is bliss. Whatever you touch is bliss. Whatever you think is bliss. Whatever movement you make is bliss. Welcome to completion stage, where you are completely bliss. You have been looking outside of yourself for bliss and peace and freedom, but you are going the wrong way. You are complete as you are, right here and right now. You are full of blissful bodhicitta.

When you feel the freedom of this blissful bodhicitta, you feel unconditional love for absolutely every being. This is not the conditional business love of unhelpfully helping family and friends and trading genital get-offs with a so-called lover. As discussed with Karmamudra, when you truly feel this level of bodhicitta, the bliss is endless, beyond this lifetime and body and self and story, and you are fully overtaken by a passion for being of benefit to all beings in whatever way, shape, and form you can across all time and space. You become the Four Immeasurables—loving kindness, compassion, joy, and equanimity—incarnate.

All the Yuthok Nyingthig practices lead to the two wings of wisdom and compassion. In Tummo Yoga, the feminine of wisdom is the red solar flame and the masculine of compassion is the white lunar drop. The flame burns the drop; the empty alchemical process releases bodhicitta; and you expand beyond ignorant self-other dualism into the freedom of Buddha Nature. It is all the same process, even as things get special and secret and sexy in terms of visualizations and energies and blah blahs.

All roads lead to Rome. That's a proverb. Now you know why I live in Rome. All roads lead to Rome—even from Tibet. All roads lead to the awakened state of Buddha Nature. The ways are different; the roads are different. Some people come on the easy road. Others, because of location, have to go across mountains, and it's difficult. Some come by walking. Some come by bicycle. Some come by motorcycle. The roads are different, and how we travel is different. But we share the destination of Rome. There is one Rome. You can come here by car or by train or by flight; it's the same. You do whatever practice floats your boat—to Rome!

Dream Yoga

Read this aloud: I am reading in my dream. I am reading in my dream. I am reading in my dream. I am reading in my dream. I am reading in my dream. I am reading in my dream. I am reading in my dream.

This is the daytime Dream Yoga practice. From time to time, during the day, you tell yourself that you are dreaming. Are you surprised to hear there is daytime Dream Yoga? Did you think Dream Yoga was only for nighttime? Did you think you only dream when you are sleeping? Did you not know you are dreaming right now?

You know how you get lost in a dream and think everything is real? You take everything in the dream so seriously! Then you wake up and feel foolish that you didn't realize it was only a dream, and you feel relieved that it was only a dream. Well, the same thing happens with your thoughts when you are awake. You think thoughts about yourself and others in your fantasies, worries, plans, memories. You take your thoughts so seriously! Just as you wake up from your dreams, you can wake up from your thoughts. You can stop being a victim of your dreams, and you can stop being a victim of your thoughts.

So there is daytime Dream Yoga to help you master your life. The process is simple but profound. From time to time, you tell yourself that you are dreaming. While you are eating, you say, "I am eating in my dream." You say this aloud seven times. You can do it with anything… I am dressing in my dream. I am walking in my dream. I am sitting in my dream. I am talking in my dream. I am listening in my dream. I am writing in my dream… It is a mindfulness practice. In mindfulness practice, people are instructed to remind themselves of what they are doing in the present moment. This is like that, but you add "in my dream." You can even say, "I am inhaling in my dream. I am exhaling in my dream."

You also do this with your emotions throughout the day. I am angry in my dream. I am proud in my dream. I am horny in my dream. I am jealous in my dream. I am scared in my dream. I am anxious in my dream. I am depressed in my dream.

You also do this with your senses. I smell rain in my dream. I hear ravens in my dream. I feel cold in my dream. I see mountains in my dream. I taste honey in my dream.

You also do this with your thoughts. I am thinking about what to make for dinner in my dream. I am considering buying a new coat in my dream. I am fantasizing about sex in my dream. I am wondering if I should text my ex in my dream.

You also let yourself know that the things around you are dream things. This is a dream book. This is a dream computer. This is a dream flower. This is a dream house. This is a dream tiramisu.

Whatever you are doing in daytime Dream Yoga, be sure to say the sentence aloud seven times. You need to repeat it because otherwise you will get distracted, like all humans. You tell yourself what is happening in your dream, and then your mind wanders off to wherever. It happens like this with any mindfulness practice. So you need to say the sentence aloud seven times. Your voice helps you to be more mindful. And if this practice doesn't make sense, you can start with, "I am confused in my dream."

However, there are some important contraindications for this practice. As is the case with any powerful medicine, do not do daytime Dream Yoga when you are operating heavy machinery or even near heavy machinery. Never ever do daytime Dream Yoga when you are driving a car or riding a bicycle or anything like that. Never ever do daytime Dream Yoga when you are in any physically risky situation, like hiking on peaks or swimming alone or anything like that. Never ever do daytime Dream Yoga when you are using a weapon or using something that could be a weapon or doing anything where you could put yourself or others in any danger. Also, do not explore daytime Dream Yoga if you have a history of dissociation or psychosis or anything like that. If you are even remotely inclined to disconnect from the reality of this physical world and your physical body, this is not the practice for you. There are many practices, so please let this one go. It is not your medicine.

On that note, though it sounds easy and seems fun, it is important to take daytime Dream Yoga very seriously because it is one of the strongest medicines on the market. You must have the foundation of Ngöndro, Guru Yoga, Tummo Yoga, and Illusory Body Yoga in order to safely explore daytime Dream Yoga. Further, like any strong medicine, it is to be prescribed while you are under the supervision of a doctor, in this case your teacher.

In its potency, daytime Dream Yoga can quite quickly shift your experience of life. Normally, when everything is happening in your life, your brain says, "This is happening; this is real. I see people, and they are real. I see trees, and they are real." Then, thanks to dualistic ignorance, we take what is relatively real and mistake it for ultimately real. Everything becomes very solid and very serious. Life becomes very heavy and very concrete. Fire types tend to have a business-oriented mind. With fire imbalance, you know all too well how to smelt what is mercurial into something solid, serious, heavy, and concrete. Living with this rigidity is not only stressful but also unnatural. There is no space, no breath, no presence. There is no awareness of the interdependence and emptiness of it all. With daytime Dream Yoga, you rebalance to become more open and flexible like wind and water. Each time you tell yourself you are in your dream, you have a different feeling than your ordinary feeling. Everything becomes illusory feeling. As with Illusory Body Yoga, you feel free of the Eight Worldly Concerns; you are liberated from hope and fear.

Daytime Dream Yoga is also preparation for nighttime Dream Yoga where you become lucid in your dreams. This means you know you are dreaming when you are dreaming. You catch the dream—you realize you are dreaming. Then you transform the dream—you do whatever you want within the dream. Cultivating awareness and agency in your dream life helps you cultivate awareness and agency in your waking life. Through Illusory Body Yoga and Dream Yoga, you understand the ultimate illusory nature of life, which means you are no longer a victim of the relative world. Of course, because of your foundation in Ngöndro and Guru Yoga, you seek to have such mastery over your life in order to be of benefit to all beings—only this altruistic motivation will unlock the door of the practice. Moreover, Dream Yoga will help you master your path in the post-death bardo so you can take rebirth into a life that allows you to be of benefit to all beings.

To catch and transform your nighttime dreams, you set yourself up for success as you go to sleep. It is best to sleep on your right side for this practice. Sleeping on your left side puts some pressure on your heart and can result in disturbing dreams. That said, sleeping on your right side is not great for digestion, so it helps to have some time between eating and sleeping. But if a teacher or doctor has told you to sleep on your left side, then please do that. You can visualize yourself as a buddha or deity, if you would like. Then you say a prayer to Yuthok, or another guru, asking for help with this practice. Then Yuthok, or another guru, descends into your throat chakra and becomes a red buddha on top of a red lotus. You can visualize this red buddha alone or in union. Or you can visualize a red flower. Or you can visualize a red light. Go with whatever works for you. There is a brief mantra—OM A NU TA RA—which you repeat, as red light radiates from the buddha, and everything becomes red and luminous, including you. The red buddha in your throat is the buddha of infinite light. Your throat chakra is the energetic center of speech and breath and light. Through this practice, you learn that everything is ultimately light in varying degrees of density. Regardless of how solid things seem to your human senses, everything is perfectly pure light.

It takes practice to become lucid in your dreams. This is because you have been practicing unawareness in both your dream life and waking life for a very long time. On that note, your dreams are usually a manifestation of your waking life in some form. The emotional tone of your dreams lets you know how your mind is really doing. Often the stress you repress during the day comes out in your dreams. But do not worry about having nice dreams to do this practice. In fact, scary dreams are sometimes easier to catch. This is called a rough catch. You get so scared that you wake yourself up to get out of the dream. So, on some level, you knew you were dreaming in your dream. Life is like this, too. On some level, you know you are dreaming during the day. That is why scary life experiences wake you up. Perhaps you can recall a moment of shock or fear when you felt clarity and presence. That was a rough catch in your dream of waking life.

To practice lucid dreaming, be on the lookout for that glimmer of awareness that you are dreaming. Then catch the dream! In the beginning, it is normal to only be lucid for a short time in your dream. Or, you may wake up as soon as you catch the dream. Again, it is like mindfulness practice. At first, you can only be mindful for a short time. Once you train, you can sustain mindfulness for longer periods of time. It is also like orgasm. Why is orgasm so short? Because we are not trained in orgasm. If you are trained in orgasm, your orgasm can be very long. It is also normal for lucid dreams to feel busy and active when you begin practicing. You may even feel stress and tiredness. Once you become more seasoned in lucid dreaming, you will wake up perfectly rested. Practices of any kind are often difficult at first. Be patient with yourself.

Once you catch the dream, then you transform the dream. To transform the dream, you must understand that you are always creating every aspect of your dreams, whether you are lucid or not. There is a funny story about this. There was a man who had a recurring nightmare where he was chased by a demon holding a knife. The man was so scared and always escaping from this dreadful demon. Finally, one night in his dream, the man decides he is tired of being scared and escaping. So he stops running, turns to the demon, and says, "Why are you chasing me? What do you want from me?" And the demon says, "I don't know. It's your dream." You are creating every single thing in your dreams. People will say they can't do visualization or they can't memorize and learn teachings or they can't blah blah blah. Hello? What do you do in your dreams? You create entire cities and entire worlds. You compose music and choreograph dance and make art and write novels. You conjure complex plots with all kinds of characters. You elicit emotions and senses. You travel to the far reaches of the earth and galaxy and unknown worlds. You become old and young and change genders and sexes. You become animals and spirits and insects. It is your dream. Once you catch the dream, you can do all of this intentionally. You can stop being the victim, puppet, and toy of your dreamy mental habits and instead transform the dream in any way you choose.

So you practice transforming. Fire types tend to have vivid dreams. So Dream Yoga can be a lot of fun for you. Play around as you learn how to transform the dream. Make yourself into a flower, first a red flower, then a blue flower, then a yellow flower, then an evergreen tree. Make yourself into a horse, running with freedom. Then the horse is chased by wolves. But you know this is a dream horse and these are dream wolves. The horse and wolves are your own energy. You can't be harmed, especially when you make yourself into a strong and powerful tiger. The wolves run away. You become a lion. You become a cow. You become a sheep. You become a snake. You become a mountain. You become a river. You become a cloud. You become rain. You become wind. You become you. You become two of you. You become ten of you. You become twenty million of you. You see a fire, but you know the dream fire cannot harm you. You see a tsunami, but you know the dream tsunami cannot harm you. You feel an earthquake, but you know the dream earthquake cannot harm you. You see people chasing you and attacking you and killing you, but you know this cannot really harm you. They are all light. You don't need to escape. Everything goes right through you. You are like a rainbow. Everything you see is your energy. You can think any thoughts and nothing disturbs you. There is no self-aggression. There is no self-conflict. You can think of your traumas and dramas, but they have no hold on you. You feel free from pain and problems. Everything is under your control. You are powerful. You can do anything. In your dream you are young. In your dream you are grown up. In your dream you are sick. In your dream you are old. In your dream you are dead. You see your funeral. You see you are buried. You see yourself dissolving into the earth and all the elements. Then you are back again. You are running in the light. You are running in the dark. It is the same. You fly to a huge city. There are many people there. So many people. Look at all these people. They are all your mental projection. You know they are all in your dream—people of different nationalities and ethnicities, elders and teenagers, babies and adults. All of these people live in your mind. You see them all as energy, and you know yourself as energy. You can go through solid objects. You go through walls and enter buildings. You go through clothes for sale in shops. You go through people and animals. Whatever you see, you go through. Energy goes through energy. You are made of light. There are no boundaries. There are no limitations. You want to go to Thailand; you go to Thailand. You want to go to Tibet; you go to Tibet. You want to go to Finland; you go to Finland. You want to go to Kenya; you go to Kenya. You want to go back to last year; you go there. You want to go to 100 years before you were born; you go there. You want to visit 100 years from now; you go there. You penetrate the planet and come out the other side. Then you do it again. You fly into space and walk on the moon and walk on the sun. You are unstoppable. Anything is possible. Everything is possible. You do it all again and again and again. You repeat this playful game of transforming and multiplying and traveling. This is called Dream Yoga.

Dream Yoga is the continuation of Illusory Body Yoga. You realize that not only is the object your projection but also the subject is your projection—and it is all light. Once you know your nature is light, then you can be very creative. Whatever you think, you become. No more questions. No more confusion. No more stagnation. No more obstacles. No more conditions. No more blaming others. No more not trusting yourself. You are the art and you are the artist. You are the creation and you are the creator. You are the philosophy and you are the philosopher. You unblock deep and profound freedom.

At this point, if you have established a proper foundation through Ngöndro and Guru Yoga, then you will naturally be drawn to the true purpose of Dream Yoga—bodhicitta. You will practice nighttime Dream Yoga not to have fantastical dream trips but to be of benefit to all beings. In your waking life, how many prostrations can you do in a day? In your dream life, you can multiply yourself into countless yous and do countless prostrations. In your waking life, you want to give offerings to your teachers but you feel stressed about money and don't have nice things. In your dream life, you can offer limitless riches and objects of beauty to your teachers and all the buddhas. In your waking life, you want to go on retreat but you have a job and a family. In your dream life, you can meditate for an eon in a mountain cave. In your waking life, you want to meet great teachers but they live far away. In your dream life, you can receive teachings from Yuthok and Medicine Buddha and any buddhas and teachers you so choose. In your waking life, you try to practice pure view but you get angry with your partner and frustrated with your colleagues and annoyed with strangers. In your dream life, you can transform all beings into buddhas and pay homage to them. In your waking life, you want to wake up and be of benefit, but you don't even know what any of that really means. In your dream life, you can manifest as a peaceful buddha, a wrathful buddha, any and all buddhas you want to be, and you can bring each and every being exactly the teachings they need to be liberated.

Now, through Dream Yoga, you see who and what you really are— infinite space, infinite time, infinite energy, infinite light, infinite love, infinite compassion, infinite joy, infinite equanimity. You are Buddha Nature.

Mahamudra

There are different ways to transmit the Buddhadharma. Ordinary humans are dense, so we need words to understand the teachings. Buddhas, on the other hand, enter meditation and communicate mind to mind. Great yogis and yoginis often receive teachings through symbols—signs, movements, colors. This kind of symbol is a mudra, which means gesture, and, in this context, refers to spiritual communication. Mahamudra is the big symbol, the big sign, the big slap that enlightens the yogi or yogini whose mind, speech, and body are primed for this type of transmission.

This is why discussion of Mahamudra usually involves stories of great yogis and yoginis. These stories serve to inspire and instruct the rest of us. However, the instruction is not instruction on how to practice Mahamudra; it is instruction on how to prepare for Mahamudra. The actual word instructions of Mahamudra are so simple that they are self-secret. An ordinary human can hear them, and even practice them, but won't achieve results unless the body, speech, and mind are primed for Mahamudra. Instead, these Mahamudra stories tell us how to approach practice if we are interested in pursuing awakening in this way. To that end, the stories have key themes—commitment, humility, devotion, hardship, and the moment of Mahamudra.

The commitment aspect of these stories illustrates what it means to take refuge in the Buddha, Dharma, and Sangha. Because this is the Tantric Buddhist path, the refuge commitment is demonstrated through the tireless pursuit of a true teacher. The student has tried other things, worldly and spiritual, but now they know only awakening can cure their ills. So they leave behind the same old, same old to seek out a qualified master. Since these stories are of a particular cultural time and place, the yogis usually have to leave high posts as rulers or scholars, including roles as Buddhist scholars, to find their teacher and receive the keys to the kingdom of enlightenment. Whereas the yoginis usually have to escape arranged marriages, and a life of comfortable-but-confining caretaking, to find their teacher and practice with abandon. Regardless of our specific circumstances in this time and place, these stories emphasize that actual practice means leaving behind conditioned ways of thinking, speaking, and doing. We must say goodbye to patterned habits of hiding and addictive forms of avoidance and comfort zones of control. We must release reactions of ignorance, desire, anger, jealousy, and pride. In other words, we must leave the bonsai pot for the forest—for good.

These stories then teach the importance of humility in Tantric Buddhism, usually through the hidden aspect of the teacher. The enlightened masters in these stories are not found on gilded thrones. They are common people doing seemingly mundane things. There is a merchant making arrows. There is a savvy businesswoman selling sesame oil and serving as a madam for prostitutes. There is a fisherman eating the stinky, discarded intestines of fish. There is a farmer with a large family and a taste for beer. Even better, these teachers often insist that they are not teachers and have nothing to show these students who pursue them relentlessly for years. And the students are hapless and flawed like the rest of us. They have gotten lost in addiction. They are totally lazy. They get distracted by pretty things. They lie to the teacher. They have even committed murder. They are messy in all the ways humans are messy, but they still find a way to meditate and get enlightened. This is an important part of Tantric Buddhism—it is open to everyone. No matter your nationality, ethnicity, race, sex, gender, sexual orientation, sexuality, income, job, habits, addictions, afflictions, there is always a way for you to wake up. After all, there is no certainty in life. Rich become poor, and poor become rich. Sick ones live long, and healthy ones die early. Life is up and down. To be a true practitioner, you need to be flexible and humble, start where you are and work with what you have.

In these stories, the students have the wish-fulfilling jewel of devotion to a teacher. To practice Mahamudra, you need a devoted relationship with a teacher who passes along the teachings to you. The big slap is a living transmission. Without a trusted teacher, your practice becomes a lot of "I'm meditating" and "I'm studying" and "I need this space" and "I'm doing this retreat" and all that I, I, I is a big obstacle. These days, a lot of people don't like to hear about devotion because it sounds too religious. But devotion is beyond religion. Maybe it is better to understand devotion as gratitude. You want to follow this path and you need help to do it, so you are overwhelmed with gratitude when you find someone who can actually show you the way. You can deepen and expand your devotion and gratitude by meditating on the miraculous interdependence of everyone and everything that has brought you here to this path—from Medicine Buddha to Yuthok to Sumtön Yeshé Zung to all the lineage masters to your teachers to your family and friends to air, water, food, and shelter. But, above all else, it is Yuthok who deserves your devotion as he has created this accessible tantric path for you to practice. Without Yuthok, you would be wandering aimlessly in the forest.

Commitment, humility, and devotion all help the students endure significant hardships on the path. The great yogis and yoginis often struggle with physical labor or risky feats or unbearable living situations, and it all seems endless and pointless. There are towers built and destroyed and built again. There are countless sesame seeds pressed for oil. There are freezing caves with terrifying storms and spirits. There are even life-threatening accidents endured. It is easy to be critical of the teachers and wonder why they put students through such physical and dangerous trials. But masters do not see students with ordinary eyes. Masters see students with the wisdom eye. Masters can see what will purify a student's karma—what will help the student get out of their own way so the teachings can be put into practice. Often these hardships are physical because that may be the fastest way to undo the energetic knots creating the toxins of afflictive emotions. In my experience, whenever students complain that the higher practices are not working, it is a sign that they have not done enough Ngöndro—especially prostrations, mandala offerings, and circumambulations—and Guru Yoga. All in all, these Mahamudra stories are offering entertaining, relatable, and varied depictions of Ngöndro and Guru Yoga through tales of hardship and devotion.

Eventually, the student receives the teachings. They learn the practices to be with the mind at rest, the mind in motion, and the nature of mind. But then comes the true moment of Mahamudra, the rough catch, the big slap when the student receives an emotional shock as awakening. Because the great yogis and yoginis have trained enough to experience emotions as pure energy, they transform emotional waves into wings of enlightenment. If you are still experiencing emotional waves as sadness and anger and anxiety and jealousy and longing, and you want to cry and fight and drink and act out and blah blah blah, then Mahamudra is not working yet. There is still more training to be done. Once you develop your mind, speech, and body for Mahamudra, then the guru of life will graciously deliver emotional waves to wake you up. You detox the toxins through transformation. Anger is the big slap of clarity.

DEDICATION

At the end of all Tantric Buddhist practices, it is customary to say a dedication prayer. Generally speaking, this prayer dedicates your practice to be of benefit to all beings. In this lineage, you request that this practice helps you quickly achieve the same enlightened state as Yuthok, and through this may you bring all beings into this state of enlightenment.

Without the dedication prayer, your practice is like a drop of water that falls in the dirt and dries up. With the dedication prayer, your practice is like a drop of water that falls in the ocean and continues to be of benefit evermore.

On that note, thank you for reading this chapter. Regardless of whether you explore this spiritual path, may the commentary on these practices be of great benefit to you and all those you encounter. May you be well and rest easy. May you shine through life like the bright light you are.

"Altruism is the most powerful
obstacle eliminator."

- Dr. Nida Chenagtsang

Chapter Five – Earth / Water

Recall a time when you were alone in nature. You were sitting or walking. Your mind was busy with this or that. Then you noticed the stability of the earth beneath you. Maybe you felt the sensation of your feet contacting dirt. Maybe you felt the sensation of your seat steady on a rock. Maybe your mind stopped for a moment because you felt grounded. Or maybe you were in a body of water. Maybe you were swimming and then turned onto your back to float. Maybe your body stopped for a moment because you felt held. Or maybe you have experienced the magic of being with our world where her mediums meet; your body supported by sand and your mind washed by waves. Maybe there you stumbled upon space.

Earth and water give us stability. They are our mother. They feed us, bathe us, and shelter us from the storm. With earth/water in our being, we are quiet, relaxed, and calm. We are gentle, patient, and dependable. Confident but modest, we get the job done in an unassuming way that is refreshing in a performative culture. We are emotionally stable and generally unfazed, which helps us hold space for our and others' emotions. Our bodies reflect this strength. Tall and solid, we are here with the big hug to wash it all away. A hug made only more delicious by our ample curves and lustrous hair, befitting the mermaids we actually are. Fortunate is the wind or fire type to enter into relationship with us as we take the edge off their volatility. We are here for the slow burn—the long, leisurely conversations with open, easy pauses that build a steady, solid connection. We know how to rest and go deep—savoring the meal, contemplating the question, taking in the view, sinking into sleep.

Similarly, in our physiology, earth/water gives us a strong and supple frame, connecting and lubricating our joints, ligaments, and bones. Our physical contraction, extension, and movement supplied by wind are all made soft and flexible by earth/water. Before fire heats up our belly to motor our digestion, it is earth/water that does the unglamorous act of breaking down and decomposing solids and liquids in our guts. But earth/water gets to have some fun as it enables sensory gratification. Earth/water allows our senses to have their rich and full experiences, giving us a feeling of satiation and satisfaction with our physical exploration of the world.

When earth/water is imbalanced, we shift from slow and supple to stuffed and stuck. We grind to a halt. Even if you are not an earth/water type, you need to pay attention to earth/water imbalance because we live in a world of distractions trying to weigh us down and pull us under and earth/water dominates childhood, which means our children are in their earth/water period. With earth/water imbalance, coldness comes over us. The coldness is deep within, first freezing up digestion, creating the backlog of constipation. To make matters worse, this coldness dampens our sense experiences, so we snack more and choose heavier, oilier meals to get some taste and pleasure, but that creates more deadweight in the gut and all over. Gradually the coldness spreads, slowing circulation, creating a chilled body and numb limbs. It is as if our entire being becomes lazy, from sticky fluids building up in the mouth and sinuses to ideas and opinions sticking around past their due date. Our contemplative conversations become monotonous monologues that lost their audience long ago. Our stability becomes conformity; our openness becomes confusion. We become lethargic and long-suffering, begrudging and stubborn, impossible to rouse from sleep, globally speaking. The mermaid sinks like a stone.

Accordingly, when your earth/water element is imbalanced, your primary mental toxin is ignorance. Mother earth/water delivers the mother of all poisons. With your mind, energy, and body feeling soggy, sluggish, and stagnant, you contract into yourself, creating the closed door of dualism from which all toxins grow. Indeed, it is ignorance that is at the root of desire and anger and all the rest. You become a black hole, sucking in life yet totally spaced out. Of course, you feel sad and stuck. Earth and water make mud.

When the poison is ignorance, what is the medicine? It is fasting. Rather than closing off in distractions, you open up with awareness. You explore less-is-more across mind, energy, and body to discover a spring in your step. Once you crack through the thick husk of ignorance, there is a spacious and easy quality to your entire being. Of course, you can fast through diet, and you may already be dreading what that means, but it will be better than you think. But you can also fast through lifestyle. And you can even fast through spiritual practice. When you fast in a fulfilling way, you are balanced. And you feel open. From that balance and openness, you can offer earth/water's spacious presence to be of benefit to us all.

DIET AND LIFESTYLE

Here is the diet-and-lifestyle pith instruction for earth/water types: Put down your phone. Put on some tunes. Sing your heart out. Dance like nobody's watching. Or, better yet, do all of that with someone you want to be watching! Then take a hot bath, have some warm soup, read a good book, and enjoy your sleep.

Earth/water types, and those with earth/water imbalance, thrive with a warm and active lifestyle. This means you do well in warm, dry, and bright places, and you do well with the warmth of physical movement and social connection. Imbalance of earth/water wants to pull you into a sedentary sinkhole of screens and snacks and sadness. So think of fasting as flowing—get up, get out, get moving. Even though you naturally might sleep the morning away, you do fine with a little less sleep, like seven hours. Setting the alarm clock for a daily group fitness class or a little outdoor adventure would start your day with a big dose of vitamin flow. Vigorous physical activity does wonders for earth/water. Think hiking, boxing, weight lifting, martial arts, and dancing. Dancing can be especially delightful with its playfulness and socializing. Yoga is also great for earth/water, but don't get stuck only doing restorative yoga. There are dynamic Tibetan yogas that can really warm you up—more on that later. You can handle a long workday of eight to nine hours, and you can handle physical labor. Be sure to spend free time in the warm glow of friends and family, even better if you take an evening walk together. While you love to learn, fasting applies to your mind, too. Rather than researching this and that on your screens, it would serve you well to take a class and deep dive with group discussion. That way learning doesn't become another solitary, addictive distraction. It must be said again that hot baths are your friend, and you can use hot salt compresses on any part of you that feels cold and stagnant.

As part of your fasting and flowing lifestyle, you do well with hot, spicy, and light food. Keep your internal waters warm with hot water, ginger tea, green and black tea, and maybe a little coffee. You do well with dried or cooked vegetables, rather than raw vegetables. Here are a few that are particularly helpful for you—radish, horseradish, leafy greens, alliums, carrots, winter squashes, peas, corn, nettle, seaweed, rhubarb, tomatoes, peppers, and chili peppers. For fruits, you do well with apples, pears, plums, dates, pomegranates, papayas, pineapple, and citrus fruits. For grains and legumes, good options are rice, barley, buckwheat, oats, quinoa, chickpeas, lentils, and beans. For meats, you do well with fish, seafood, mutton, lamb, pork, yak, beef, duck, chicken, and rabbit. Olive oil, sesame oil, ghee, sunflower oil, walnut oil, yogurt, buttermilk, butter, and plant-based dairy alternatives should work for you. You want spices that warm your belly, so try chili pepper, cumin, mustard, anise, cinnamon, cardamom, salt, and, your good friend, ginger.

As for fasting, in general, it would serve you well to stick to whole foods and regular meals that satisfy without stuffing you. Eat until almost full, not overfull. And try to cut down on sugar, which ruins the already sweet soil of earth/water's gut garden. As for actual fasting, if it works for your mind and energy, you can take a meal off now and then, at most once per day. You could have some warm tea or hot broth instead. A fun fact is the Buddha was a proponent of intermittent fasting, in his own way. Maybe you have heard that the Buddha's sangha received all of their food from the surrounding community. The sangha would walk each day with their bowls and take whatever the community had to offer. In the spirit of non-attachment, the Buddha told his sangha to accept and eat everything offered to them. And, in the spirit of non-stress, he made no demands on the community, allowing them to fill the bowls with whatever they had to offer. Of course, this led to some difficult-to-digest meals for the sangha. So the Buddha instructed his sangha to only eat twice a day— breakfast and lunch. This gave their digestive systems the necessary space to process whatever came their way. You, too, can give your system a little space by fasting for a meal or eating lightly when possible. You can also use hot water as medicine to move things along. You can experiment with what helps you to feel your best.

For earth/water types, this is an interesting contemplation—what does it feel like to feel your best? Unfortunately, you may not even know. When the poison is ignorance, the addiction is numbing. You tune out the experience of being alive, usually through binging—food, sweets, tech, weed, whatever it takes. The thing is, shoving things down shuts you down. Because when you numb, you don't just numb the negative, you numb it all. You become zombie-like, going through the motions. So fasting serves as a reboot to feel again, starting with genuine hunger. A healthy and honest hunger leads people to make nourishing choices— around food, media, technology, relationships, work, sex, everything. You need space to know what you truly want. Fasting is not meant to punish or shame you, not at all. Fasting is meant to give you a fighting chance to feel alive. From there, you can choose how you want to live.

SPIRITUAL PRACTICE

Now we will transition into spiritual medicine for earth/water. You might think fasting as a spiritual practice means extreme renunciation or austerities, but it is actually subtler than that. On this tantric path, fasting means finding the fine line between spaciousness and spacing out. To that end, we will look at Ngöndro practices, pre-empowerment practices, and post-empowerment practices of Guru Yoga/creation stage and completion stage—all with a focus on fasting and balancing earth/water. Please note that what follows is a unique commentary on these practices. Of course, there is some instruction within the commentary. However, to practice Ngöndro, Guru Yoga, creation stage, and completion stage, you need a teacher to give you a reading transmission of the root text along with practice instructions. For now, you can explore the potential of these practices from the perspective of fasting and balancing to consider how the Yuthok Nyingthig could help you be of benefit to yourself and others.

NGÖNDRO

Refuge

Buddha means awakened one. Taking refuge in the Buddha means taking refuge in waking up. This means being present. We hear this term "being present" so much that it is losing its meaning. What does it mean to wake up and be present? One of my sons used to watch a reality-television show called *Naked and Afraid*. Maybe you have heard of it? People are dropped off in a remote location to survive in the wilds of nature, and they do this naked. No more bonsai pot for them! I like the title of this show—*Naked and Afraid*. I like the title in Italian even more—*Nudi e Crudi*. It means naked and raw. Being present is being naked and raw—with your experience. This does not mean feeling sad or happy, and then labeling yourself as sad or happy, and then journaling about being sad or happy, and then telling everyone about being sad or happy. It means feeling the mental, energetic, and physical experience of feelings without adding any labels. You stop layering your experience with stories. You stop filtering your experience through concepts. You experience your experience—naked and raw.

Earth/water types tend to have an abundant nature. You like to take in the world. In perfect balance, your openness to life lends itself to taking refuge in naked and raw experience. As such, earth/water types tend to be drawn to tantra with its acceptance of sensory delights. Having found an alternative to the seemingly bare-bones approach of sutra, you are thrilled to take refuge in a path that allows for the richness of humanness. But perfect balance is hard to come by. So, usually, the wisdom of opening distorts into the ignorance of insulating. You literally take in the world—stuffing yourself however you can. And now, with tantra, you think you have a green light to do so. You don't need to deny yourself anything; you just need to do it all dharma style. You stuff your brain with dharma books. You stuff your home with dharma statues. You stuff your days with dharma talks. You stuff your calendar with dharma retreats. You stuff your plate with dharma feasts. You stuff your belly with dharma meat. You stuff your anxiety with dharma alcohol. You stuff your genitals with dharma sex. You stuff your ego with dharma names. This is not waking up. This is numbing with spiritual shit.

So the challenge for you, good earth/water one, is to explore the fasting of refuge. There is a big difference between taking refuge in the Buddha and getting lost in the trappings of Buddhism. Being on the tantric path just means you take refuge in the naked and raw experiences that come with whatever hand life has dealt you, like your job and your family. Tantra was designed to be pragmatic, not sexy—that nonsense is all contemporary marketing. On that note, taking refuge in the Dharma does not mean creating a new dharma life full of dharma experiences and dharma display. You just take refuge in the truths presented in the teachings—noting the impermanence and suffering in everyday life, and bringing the wisdom of emptiness along with the maturity of compassion and the sanity of a middle way without extreme views to whatever you happen to be doing, like going to the grocery store. Likewise, taking refuge in the Sangha does not mean finding all new sangha people, especially in tantra. Your family and coworkers and strangers at the grocery store are all humans on the path of life with you—there's your sangha; respect them and learn from them. And, if you do have a community of peers on your spiritual path, same thing applies—whoever shows up, respect them and learn from them. Taking refuge is really about simplifying your life. Nudi e crudi.

Bodhicitta

In its clarifying of purpose, bodhicitta is a big dose of fasting. While it is customary to say the Bodhicitta prayer at the start of formal practice, it would be balancing for you to do a brief, internal call-and-response before any dharma-related activity. Why am I doing this? To be of benefit to all beings.

Why am I reading this dharma book? To be of benefit to all beings.
Why am I listening to this dharma podcast? To be of benefit to all beings.
Why am I doing this dharma practice? To be of benefit to all beings.
Why am I here on this dharma retreat? To be of benefit to all beings.

This will help you on two levels. First, bodhicitta cuts through the muck. As you walk this spiritual path, your natural abundance could mean that you accumulate a lot of blah blah blah about why, when, and how you are doing what you are doing. Let bodhicitta blast it all out of your mind. If you are practicing this Tantric Buddhist path, your purpose is to be of benefit to all beings. With that simple and clear motivation, watch how simple and clear your practice can become. Instead of drowning in dharma dos and don'ts, dharma plans and props, dharma rules and regulations, dharma dress and drama, just do your dharma practice to be of benefit to all beings. Fasting is refreshing like that.

Also, bodhicitta cracks through your crust. The imbalanced insulating energy of earth/water may lead you to isolate. You keep your spiritual life private and precious. You practice alone in a comfort zone of control. When you separate yourself, physically and/or emotionally, from the rest of us, your spirituality becomes dry and theoretical and you become detached and academic. You lose the juice of love. The more you stir up your love of all beings through bodhicitta, the more you will open yourself to being with all beings. Next thing you know, you are enjoying all beings. Even better, you find yourself doing everything you do to be of benefit to all beings. Generosity, morality, effort, patience, meditation, and wisdom become your way of being. When you clarify your purpose through bodhicitta, you clearly display your open heart—and it feels wonderful. I had a student who was experiencing chronic pain, and her days were filled with personal healing, personal treatments, and personal spirituality. And none of it was working. The only time she didn't feel pain was when she was practicing Ngöndro—bodhicitta broke through it all.

The Four Immeasurables

Focusing on the Four Immeasurables prayer is perfect for fasting. The entire path can be boiled down to the Four Immeasurables. So please let the Four Immeasurables be your cup of hot broth when the dharma feels difficult to digest.

The Four Immeasurables prayer in the Yuthok Nyingthig is a series of sentences that are spoken and contemplated:

> *May all beings have happiness and the causes of happiness.*
> *May all beings be free from suffering and the causes of suffering.*
> *May all beings never be separated from the supreme joy*
> *that is beyond all suffering.*
> *May all beings abide in equanimity, free from attachment,*
> *aversion, and sorrow.*

For wind imbalance, as a medicine of nourishment, we applied the Four Immeasurables to oneself and then to all those we want to help. For fire imbalance, as a medicine of detoxing, we applied the Four Immeasurables to all those we find difficult, especially those who stir our anger. But there is another group to consider in our prayers, a very precious group of beings—the ones we don't notice. They will be the fasting focus for earth/water.

As discussed, when the poison is ignorance, we drown in dualism. This displays in 84,000 ways, and we have 84,000 medicines to counteract it. One antidote for dualistic ignorance is to notice all the people, animals, and insects you typically ignore throughout your day. Traditionally, in Buddhism, it is taught that all beings have been your mother at some point in your countless lives. So, as you make your way through your day, you can consider how every being you pass has birthed you, held you, fed you, rocked you to sleep, and prioritized your needs over theirs as they raised you. If that contemplation doesn't do much for you, then focus on this life now. The imbalance of earth/water can cloud your awareness, meaning you only notice and prioritize your small cocoon of concerns and pleasures. Actively noticing and considering strangers shakes you out of yourself. You don't need to strike up conversations or bother people or get up in their business. You just allow yourself to see people, really see people, and think about their existence. How is their day going? Do they have a proper place to sleep? Do they have enough food? Do they have supportive family and friends? Do they feel relaxed? Or choose one thing you worry about for yourself and consider that many others are worried about that same thing—like safety, family, finances, career, health, love, sex, friendship. Crack open your cocoon and let yourself feel the warmth of community—the community of human beings who are going through all the same things you are going through. For extra credit, you can extend this contemplation to animals. For super duper bonus, you can extend this contemplation to insects. And, if you want to get really wild, you can extend this contemplation to unseen beings who inhabit our world, like nature spirits. When you let yourself see, really see, another being, you can silently say to yourself:

> *May you have happiness and the causes of happiness.*
> *May you be free from suffering and the causes of suffering.*
> *May you never be separated from the supreme joy*
> *that is beyond all suffering.*
> *May you abide in equanimity, free from attachment,*
> *aversion, and sorrow.*

Stop stuffing yourself with your own blah blahs. Pick your head up and look around. The vast ocean of beings need not be overwhelming. Just see one and send them these good wishes. Through one being at a time, you can be in love with the world.

Prostrations

In the Southern California mountains, where we have a retreat center, they experience the threat of mudslides when there are big rains. When water can't flow, it creates thick, heavy mud that weighs down the mountain, eventually creating a slide that destroys plant and animal and even human life. One way to prevent mudslides is to keep water flowing.

Earth/water energy in a body acts the same way it does in nature. If earth/water energy does not flow, it creates toxic mud that weighs you down and destroys everything from your gut microbiome to blood circulation to emotional intelligence to sexual function. You become a constipated, frozen-limbed, grudge-holding, libido-lacking mudslide of meh. Earth/water types, and those with earth/water imbalance, need to find flow. Remember, you can think of fasting as flowing.

Prostrations are magical medicine for flow. On a physical level, the stretching and squeezing and huffing and puffing all warms and lubricates and circulates earth/water energy. This energetic balance keeps your limbs supple and flexible, your digestive pipes clean and clear, your senses open and alert, your hair thick and glossy. On an emotional level, the strenuous and dynamic motion stimulates all those happy hormones of bodhicitta, allowing you to display your strengths of stability, patience, gentleness, and kindness. On a spiritual level, the focus of the prostrations clarifies the source of your path—the teacher. Without your teacher, none of this would be possible. Again, in your abundance, you may have collected a lot of buddhas and deities and practices and promises, but the wellspring of your liberation is your teacher. Slowly slowly, the prostrations clear the clutter, fasting you into a sense of flow, where it is abundantly obvious where your true promise and gratitude lies:

From whose kindness great bliss itself instantly arises within us,
the guru with jewel-like form, holder of the vajra,
I prostrate at your feet.

Mandala

Let things go. This is how you fast through Mandala offering. You find the flow of letting things go. Specifically, you practice letting go of wounds and resentments. Earth/water types have an easygoing, dependable, and placating nature. Thanks to this combination, you are often the shelter for others' storms. People unload their emotional stuff onto you. People even place their serious pain upon you. Whether you are providing a listening ear or you are providing an easy target for someone's anger and abuse, you tend to just take it. In your gentleness, avoidance, and muddiness, you silently absorb all the stuff. And then, with your inclination toward insulation, you hold on to it. You hold on to the emotional and energetic stuff of yourself and others. From that epicenter of gripping, you might hold on to other stuff like poop and weight and things. You keep holding and holding. Over time, you become quiet and heavy in so many ways.

Until one day when you can't keep it in anymore. The earth shakes, and the dam breaks, and that is never a pretty picture.

Mandala offering can show you how to gracefully let things go. In your visualized offering, you gather whatever you want to give to your compassionate teachers and all the enlightened buddhas. Remember, their minds have gone beyond concepts of good and bad; they are happy to receive whatever you have to offer. Give them your treasures, give them your triumphs, give them your troubles, give them your traumas. Gather it. Offer it. Let it go. Along with the visualization, the practice involves saying a prayer and making a mudra—a small physical gesture of gathering, offering, letting go. As you say the prayer and move your hands, you feel the flow. Gather, offer, let it go. Gather, offer, let it go. Gather, offer, let it go. Slowly slowly, you will feel the freedom of flow.

As this process imprints in your mind, energy, and body, you will learn how to gradually and gracefully let go of what is no longer serving you. Don't rush yourself. Don't deny what has happened. Take your time to gather it and see it and know it. Offer all the lessons learned to serve the highest purpose of self and other. Then let it go. Over time, it will become increasingly instinctive to harvest the lessons but then let go of your problems and wounds and also to let go of others' problems and wounds. You will see and feel how holding on serves no one. When you generously let things go, you free yourself to be who you are now and you free others to be who they are now.

Because you are a deep thinker who likes to contemplate, consider this: The past has as much reality as the dream you had last night. Both have left hazy memories in your mind. But, thanks to emptiness, one is not more real than the other. This is also true of ten seconds ago. It has no more reality than your dream last night. What are you actually holding on to? Just as you have let go of the drama of last night's dream, you can let go of the drama of the past. You can let go of the burdens and wounds and secrets and stories and grudges and gripes. Take what helps you be of benefit and release the rest. Use your natural spaciousness to see the truth. Life is simply an ongoing process of gathering, offering, letting it go.

Circumambulation

When you imagine a Buddhist what do you see? Probably someone sitting. In the past, maybe a lot of sitting was good for Buddhists because everyone was active. The monks and nuns worked all day in the temple. The yogis and yoginis were often farmers. So they all got to finally take a break and sit down whenever they meditated.

But today our number one problem is a sedentary lifestyle. Do you sit a lot? Do you have problems? Now you know why.

Cardiovascular disease, depression, all these things that destroy us can be combatted by movement. But not too much movement. We live in a time of extremes where sporty people move too much and sitty people move too little. We need to find the middle way of movement. You know what that is? Walking. Walking is the perfect exercise because it gets you up, gets you out, and gets those happy hormones flowing, all while burning excess calories and strengthening muscles without putting too much stress and strain on your joints. It is simple and can be social and just thirty minutes a day goes a long way.

The Yuthok Nyingthig Ngöndro is unique in including circumambulations. One reason for this walking practice within Ngöndro is to maintain your health. Because this lineage has a focus on healing, attention is paid to your physical body. If you recall, Yuthok the Elder was a legendary walker. So please take circumambulations on the road. Go outside, visualize Medicine Buddha over your right shoulder, and take a vigorous walk while saying his mantra, audibly or silently—

TADYATA OM BEKADZE BEKADZE MAHA BEKADZE RADZA SAMUDGATE SOHA.

For earth/water types, it is imperative that you move. This cannot be said enough. Movement is your most important medicine for mind, energy, and body. Remember, fasting is flowing. Get your body flowing with walking. Get your speech-energy flowing with mantra. Get your mind flowing with awareness. When imbalanced, earth/water has a tendency to tune out. Use circumambulations to tune in. Tune in to your body and observe its sensations. Tune in to your energy and observe your impermanent moods. Tune in to your mind and observe its motion or stillness. Tune in to your surroundings and observe the human, animal, plant, and insect life around you. You are energetically of the earth—get out there and be with it and be with yourself and be with all that is. Watch how movement wakes you up.

Vajrasattva

In its purification, Vajrasattva practice is all about flow. People tend to think of purification as letting go of all the negative things you think, say, and do. On a basic level, this is true. There are emotional toxins that create pain in your mind, energy, and body. This pain leads to negative thoughts, speech, and actions that harm yourself and others. But another way to think of these toxins is stagnation—a blockage of flow. When there is proper flow, your mind, energy, and body stay with the present moment. You experience all you experience entirely in the now so nothing sticks. There is no residue of rumination. There is no build up of blah blahs. There is no unnecessary activity. This perspective reframes "good" as being in the present moment and "bad" as being anywhere else, like dwelling on the past or projecting into the future. When you are in the present, all is well. Maybe you have had this experience of pure presence. No matter what is happening around you or within you, when you are completely present, you are okay. Actually, you are better than okay; you are awake. When you are awake, you are able to see and offer what is needed at any time, which is usually spacious awareness. Presence is pretty much the most powerful medicine we can give self and other. So you can think of Vajrasattva's purification as a flow of presence running through your being. This is the flow of fasting—you stop chewing on what was or feasting on what will be and open to what is.

We have already discussed the basics of Vajrasattva practice. You visualize Vajrasattva—or Yuthok or another guru or a ball of light—above your head, releasing healing nectar into your crown point. You can visualize this nectar as liquid or light of any healing color. You let the nectar flow through your entire body as you say Vajrasattva's mantra, audibly or silently. As you do this, whatever you would like to release flows out from your orifices and pores. It is an energetic shower of presence.

For you, good earth/water one, it could be especially fruitful to focus on the felt sensation of nectar finding every nook and cranny of your body. When earth/water is imbalanced, we tend to feel dense, muddy, and cloudy. We lose touch with our subtle, internal energetic experience. This can happen to anyone of any typology. One sign of this loss is grasping at sense pleasures. Earth/water energy allows us to experience and enjoy our senses, but earth/water imbalance results in relentlessly seeking pleasurable sensory experiences. When you are energetically balanced and completely present, you might find that any sense experience is pleasurable. You don't need to do or seek anything special. Just being alive in the moment feels delightful. Then any amplified sense experience, like a truck reversing or an airplane passing, could bring you into bliss. To reclaim your inherent sensory sensitivity, you can purify yourself into the present with Vajrasattva. Start from your head and track the experience of nectar flowing through every bit of your being. Go at your own pace and be patient. Explore your energetic body with this healing nectar of flow.

As you fill with the flow of living, you will crowd out the stagnant stuff that has been sitting around. Your mind, energy, and body will align in the now. When you are completely present, there is nowhere for the toxins to take hold. You might find that fasting from toxins is as simple as can be.

Kusali Body Offering

These days, it is not necessarily easy to have an earth/water body. Mainstream culture mostly praises muscular fire bodies and lean wind bodies. You might only receive praise for your curvy earth/water body if your curves are in all the socially approved places or if you excel at sports requiring strength. As an earth/water type, it might be all too easy to feel badly about your body based on social blah blahs. Besides the fact that all bodies are beautiful, it would be good if people understood that the most nurturing human qualities come with earth/water energy and thus often an earth/water body. What most of us need in order to grow and heal is a steady, spacious presence—someone who can provide support without getting in the way. In other words, we need earth/water energy. Of course we do. Look around. As has been said, earth/water is our mother—our original source of growth and healing. Earth/water types need to know that their physical earth/water abundance is supporting their mental and energetic earth/water spaciousness. It is a precious and gorgeous gift you have.

In Chöd practice, you visualize your body as an offering. Your body transforms into nectar that gives every being exactly what they need in order to grow and heal. Before your body becomes an offering, you often visualize it increasing. Your body becomes a mountain and then an ocean of nectar. In other words, your body becomes earth/water and you energetically offer it to all beings.

There's a lesson here for earth/water types to embrace the entirety of your being. Maybe Chöd can be an opportunity to fast away any negative self-talk surrounding your body. After all, societal praise and approval is brought to you by the hamster wheel of suffering; let it go and find your flow. Please remember that you can bring the bounty of earth/water's nurturing and healing energy to all beings, all the time.

PRE-EMPOWERMENT PRACTICE

Eliminating Obstacles

Eliminating Obstacles is a Guru Yoga that you can do prior to receiving the Yuthok Nyingthig empowerment because it does not require you to generate as a buddha or deity. You practice this Guru Yoga as you are. It is the perfect place for earth/water types to begin because it clears anything blocking your path. The slow and accumulating energy of earth/water could create a lot of stuff between you and practice. You might have material stuff, like you need to organize your space to have a place to practice. You might have physical stuff, like body pains that need to be soothed for you to walk or sit or lie down to practice. You might have emotional stuff, like resentment or hesitation regarding practice. You might have mental stuff, like confusion about how to start practice. Whatever the case, Eliminating Obstacles helps you honor that little spark in you that wants to wake up.

For this practice, you can walk or sit or lie down. As always, you begin with Refuge, Bodhicitta, and the Four Immeasurables. Good motivation leads to good meditation—and altruism is the most powerful obstacle eliminator. For this visualization, you remain as yourself, but the nature of your body is light. You are full of light and free of physical substances like bones, muscles, or organs. Above your head is a giant four-petaled pink lotus, or you can choose whatever color you would like for the lotus. In the center of the lotus is a flat moon disc. Sitting on the moon disc is Yuthok, or your preferred guru. Yuthok has long, dark, flowing hair and is wearing a white robe, all symbolizing the uncontrived natural state. In his right hand, he is holding the arura plant just like Medicine Buddha. The arura plant represents the three fruits of dharma, wealth, and happiness. These are the three things most people look for in life: spiritual awakening, material comfort, and joy. In Yuthok's left hand, he holds a vase filled with obstacle-eliminating nectar.

As in Outer Guru Yoga, Yuthok is surrounded by the four medicine goddesses, or whatever gender and form of deity you would like. These goddesses eliminate obstacles in your ordinary life. In front of Yuthok is the white goddess playing a lute. She pacifies disturbances; for example, she cures physical ailments. To the right of Yuthok is the yellow goddess playing a flute. She increases deficiencies; for example, she boosts your energy and income. In back of Yuthok is the red goddess playing a trumpet. She controls strong emotions or situations; for example, she squashes your interest in unhealthy relationships. To the left of Yuthok is the green goddess holding a silver mirror. She destroys negativities; for example, she clears disturbing outside energies or internal stories of doubt. With these four actions of pacifying, increasing, controlling, and destroying, you can eliminate all of your mundane obstacles so that your ordinary life can be as you wish.

Then you ask Yuthok to help you achieve your spiritual wish of enlightenment. Specifically, you ask Yuthok to eliminate obstacles to your realizing your inherent Buddha Nature.

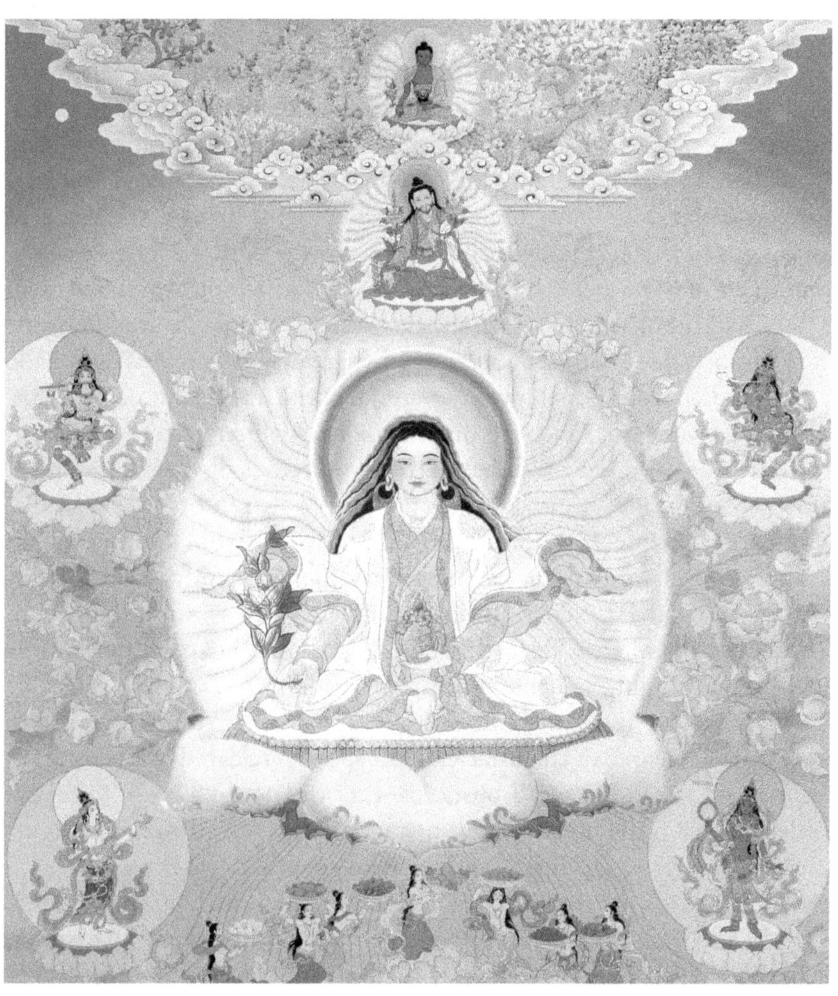

Eliminating Obstacles Yuthok

Having heard your requests, Yuthok radiates light from his head, throat, and heart—offering to all the buddhas and eliminating the obstacles of all beings. His head radiates white light. His throat radiates red light. His heart radiates blue light. Imagine and feel these lights above your crown expanding in all directions. Then rainbow light returns to Yuthok, bringing all of your favorite buddhas, deities, protectors, gurus, and teachers. Feel them all dissolving into Yuthok like snowflakes melting in the sun. Yuthok contains the blessings of all your trusted spiritual supporters, and his body becomes rainbow light. Bring a felt sense of awareness to this bright light above your crown. In that energetic space, there is a thousand-petaled lotus that will open when you are enlightened.

As Yuthok completely fills with rainbow light, so, too, does his vase of obstacle-eliminating nectar. The nectar flows up and out of the vase and then drips down into your crown point. The nectar drips, drips, drips. Take your time and feel this sensation of dripping nectar at the top of your head. You are reawakening your awareness of the energy there. Slowly the obstacle-eliminating nectar drips down into your body, like Vajrasattva practice. As the nectar flows through your body, you can say the Eliminating Obstacles mantra, audibly or silently—OM MAHA GUNA SIDDHI HUNG. Your head completely fills with rainbow light. Your throat completely fills with rainbow light. Your heart completely fills with rainbow light. Your navel completely fills with rainbow light. Your base completely fills with rainbow light. You receive Yuthok's blessings. Your body is cleared of all obstacles. Your speech is cleared of all obstacles. Your mind is cleared of all obstacles. Feel the nectar flow within you. Inner flow leads to outer flow. You can move gracefully through your life, accomplishing your ordinary and spiritual goals with ease.

To close the practice, you can ask Yuthok to bless your mind, speech, and body. You can also request that anything you think, speak, or do be medicine for yourself and others. You can then add any personal prayers. With your prayers complete, Yuthok dissolves into you. All obstacles are eliminated. Rest in this awareness.

Nejang Yoga

How's this for abundance? Earth/water types get an extra pre-empowerment practice! You may be thinking that you do not have time for many practices, but that is ignorance talking. These days, the problem is that we have too much time. We have time for depression, laziness, anxiety, conflicts, procrastination, internet, social media, and blah blah blah. Somehow, we have time for all these things that make us feel bad but no time for something that will make us feel good. To jumpstart earth/water energy back into balance, it helps to have extra options. Because moving is essential to flowing, it would be wonderful if you could practice yoga.

The Tibetan word for yoga can be translated as returning to your primordial humanness. Yoga renews your connection with your original state. Without this internal connection, you will keep looking externally for connections. You will find things you like; you will find things you don't like; and then that will all change. There is no end to external searching, and it never works. Yoga creates a bridge back to your uncontrived state. In other words, it brings you back to the forest.

To that end, there is a particular Tibetan yoga that serves as a self-healing practice. It is called Nejang Yoga—and it is beneficial for everyone of every typology. Nejang Yoga can be translated as purifying the places. There are twenty-four energy locations in the human body that get clogged up. Again, you can think of toxins as stagnation. Through this yoga practice of breath retention, gentle movement, and self-massage, you can recycle the toxins into remedies. Essentially, Nejang Yoga is a dose of medicinal flow. You can make Nejang Yoga as relaxed or as intense as you would like. It is mostly performed seated, and it is accessible for anyone in any condition. I wrote a brief book about Nejang Yoga that provides an explanation of the practice as well as instructions on how to do the practice. It is called *Nejang: Tibetan Self-Healing Yoga*. There are also certified Nejang Yoga teachers worldwide. Please do give it a try. It can transform us all back into organic, living, breathing human beings.

Three-Part Purification Breathing

When you are shut down and confused and closed off, what kind of animal are you? Are you a sloth? Are you a flounder? Are you a chicken? Now imagine your ignorance as that animal. Choose whatever animal you would like.

Then prepare to release that animal from your being and with it all of your ignorance. You can do this through a three-part breathing exercise. Take a smooth inhale, gently retain the breath for a moment, and on the exhale visualize a zillion of your ignorance animals leaving the body through all of your orifices and pores. So long, sloths. Farewell, flounders. Ciao, chickens. Smooth inhale, gentle retention, exhale the animals. If you want a sound to go with it, silently say "OM" on the inhale, "AH" on the retention, and "HUNG" on the exhale. If you want a color to go with it, visualize white light entering you on the inhale, red light spreading through you on the retention, and blue light leaving you with the animals on the exhale. Or choose other soothing sounds and colors. Or use the sounds and colors but not the animal visualization. Do it whenever you want or as a formal practice for a few minutes each day. Don't overthink it.

Mantra Healing

As mentioned, mantra, or mind protection, is a form of self-therapy. To fast with mantra, flow with it. Say it quickly, over and over again. You could set an accumulation goal for yourself and try to do a certain number each day. You can count your repetitions with a mala or a small counter or your fingers. Mantra repetition can warm you up and get you in gear. A simple and powerful mantra is OM AH HUNG, which was suggested for the breathing exercise above. You can start there and see how it goes.

POST-EMPOWERMENT PRACTICE – CREATION STAGE

Concise Guru Yoga

Concise Guru Yoga gets to the heart of the matter—opening your heart chakra. We have talked about how all buddhas are in one buddha and all gurus are in one guru. This goes for chakras as well. If you truly open one chakra, the rest will flower open. This is especially true with the heart chakra. When you open the heart chakra, it opens the door of infinite space. This is the final wake-up call.

In the Yuthok Nyingthig, the four Guru Yogas work together to support your path of awakening. The intended process is to practice Outer Guru Yoga, Inner Guru Yoga, and Secret Guru Yoga as seven-day retreats, and also daily practices, before turning to the ongoing daily practice of

Concise Guru Yoga. However, in its simplicity, Concise Guru Yoga could be the best fit for earth/water types, and those with earth/water imbalance, if you are procrastinating and need to streamline your spiritual practice. Also, in the spirit of fasting, Concise Guru Yoga contains the essential elements of all the Guru Yogas—you get a lot of bang for your buck. So, if you feel overwhelmed by the thought of multiple Guru Yogas, jump in with Concise Guru Yoga and see what happens. A nice daily practice session could be Eliminating Obstacles followed by Concise Guru Yoga. Again, because Concise Guru Yoga is a creation stage practice, it requires proper transmission and instruction, but we can discuss the basics here to put you in the mood.

As always, please recite Refuge, Bodhicitta, and the Four Immeasurables at the start of practice to establish an altruistic motivation and proper foundation. For Concise Guru Yoga, you generate as Medicine Buddha. In fact, you generate as fancy Medicine Buddha. Often, in the Yuthok Nyingthig, when generating as Medicine Buddha, the instruction is to generate as Medicine Buddha in simple form. This means a basic robe and no jewelry, all symbolizing freedom from craving. But, in Concise Guru Yoga, you generate as Medicine Buddha in the enjoyment body. This means fancy robes along with jeweled bracelets and necklaces and earrings, all symbolizing an embrace of the sense pleasures. Rather than refusing or escaping the senses, you use them as an opportunity for meditation. You embody enjoyment. This is another reason why Concise Guru Yoga works well for earth/water types; you are naturally drawn to enjoyment, so you are invited to use it as a path of awakening. As Medicine Buddha, you are holding the arura plant in your right hand. We discussed how the arura plant represents the three fruits of dharma, wealth, and happiness. You can also think of these fruits as physical enlightenment, speech-energy enlightenment, and mental enlightenment. As Medicine Buddha, you are also holding a bowl of healing nectar in your left hand. As always, you are made of light like a hologram—in this case, the healing blue light of Medicine Buddha.

With Concise Guru Yoga, you don't visualize anything above your head or within all the chakras. Again, you go straight to the heart of the matter—your heart. In your heart, you visualize a blue lotus. On top of this lotus is a vajra that radiates light, offering to all the buddhas, which of course includes all of your favorite buddhas, deities, gurus, and teachers. Drawn to the light, they bring their blessings to you and dissolve into the vajra in your heart like snowflakes melting in the sun. Supercharged with spiritual support, you then offer light from the vajra in your heart to all beings. This light brings all beings happiness and the causes of happiness. This light eliminates all of their suffering. This light gives them endless joy. This light is equanimity. Remember to send this light to all beings—not only those who elicit your affection and aversion but also the unnoticed beings of your world. Having brought benefit to all beings, the light returns to your heart, and the vajra transforms into the guru Yuthok.

Yuthok is in the center of your heart, blue in color and sitting upon the blue lotus. And he is not alone. He is in union with a fiery-red female deity. As always, feel free to change the genders and colors to whatever suits you. Both of them are in their enjoyment bodies, wearing jeweled ornaments, and deeply energized and alive with connection.

He is holding a vajra and a vase of long-life nectar. She is holding a white skull cup full of blood symbolizing the union of wisdom and compassion. She is also holding a curved knife. This knife is eliminating four demons. The first demon is death, which marks an end to this life's precious opportunity to practice. The second demon is the mental, energetic, and physical components of this embodied life of suffering. The third demon is your habitual poisons of ignorance, anger, and desire, which will propel you into your next life of suffering. The fourth demon is temporary enjoyment.

The demon of temporary enjoyment includes all of your addictions. Maybe you get lost in drugs or alcohol. When you take these substances, you escape into pleasurable sensation. But then without these substances, you feel down and nonfunctional and needing to take them again. Or maybe your demon is food. Or maybe your demon is clothes. Or maybe your demon is cars. Or maybe your demon is decorating. Or maybe your demon is vacations. Or maybe your demon is lovers. Or maybe your demon is media. Or maybe your demon is technology. Whatever temporary enjoyment distracts you from the present moment, it has a demonic force because it is separating you from awakening, not to mention controlling you and giving you problems. This is tricky though isn't it—to tell you to visualize buddhas in their enjoyment bodies and then tell you enjoyment is a demon. So the invitation is for you to discern between temporary enjoyment and transcendent enjoyment. Concise Guru Yoga can release you from temporary fixes to find transcendent freedom. All you have to do is show up and get out of the way. Stop being your own obstacle and do the practice.

Having established these two buddhas in union in your heart, the heart of Concise Guru Yoga is a mantra exchange between them. You visualize a mantra chain of light going from one buddha to the other, first at the mouth, then at the genitals, over and over again. This creates flowing light in your heart, which opens your heart chakra.

With continued practice, you come to know the nature of your heart, which is the nature of your mind. Slowly slowly, you feel a sense of union in your heart/mind. We are not talking about the superficial sexual union of the buddhas—that is only a symbol. We are talking about an indivisible union with everyone and everything. This is not static oneness but dynamic wholeness. It is like twilight, the ungraspable union of light and dark. This is the awakening of emptiness in your heart/mind.

With the arousal of emptiness comes a sensation of great bliss. These days, people blah blah about full-body orgasms, trying to start such things from rubbing their genitals. But the big orgasm, the great orgasm, the transcendent orgasm, is your heart orgasm. And this orgasm is bringing you much more than pleasure and bliss. It is bringing you into complete bodhicitta—loving kindness, compassion, joy, and equanimity. In your wholeness, you become nothing but limitless loving space.

Through Concise Guru Yoga, there is a flow from the enjoyment body into the body of infinite space. And there is a lesson here for earth/water types. Yes, the sense pleasures are embraced on this path. Yes, your humanness is affirmed. But the senses are doors, not destinations. Don't get stuck in the demon of temporary joy. Find the flow of transcendent joy. Lighten your touch. The ethereal union of bliss-emptiness awaits.

POST-EMPOWERMENT PRACTICE – COMPLETION STAGE

Tummo Yoga

To truly journey from the enjoyment body into the infinite-space body, you need to deal with your physical body. Have you ever seen the contents of a human? Maybe if you are a doctor you have had the privilege of seeing a human body cut open. Or maybe you have had the misfortune of being in or near an accident and seen the same. If so, you know that the human body is meat. It looks just like the dead animal bodies you see on the side of the road or for sale at the butcher. We like to show our skin and flex our muscles, but it is all just meat. What do you think reincarnation means? You come back as carne. You come back as meat. The problem is you get stuck inside this meat, and then you become dense. The meat and mind become numb and dumb. You think this meat is all there is. You feed the meat and flaunt the meat and diet the meat and drug the meat and sex the meat and selfie the meat. This is not living as an organic human. This is living as a zoned-out zombie. Even if you look pretty as a picture, you are going through the motions as meat. You are no different than the meat at the grocery store—cold, compartmentalized, and covered in plastic.

Tummo fire is the antidote to your zombie existence. Hello? Zombies? You need to heat your meat. This means you need to move your meat. In tantra, you are not only working with your mind; you are also working with your body. Again, tantra means body protection. In the previous chapter on fire energy, we focused on the enlightening power of tummo fire and Tummo Yoga. So please be sure to read that section. As discussed, the Yuthok Nyingthig Tummo Yoga has three components—visualization, breathing, and physical exercises. Whereas fire types may need to back off from the physical exercises because of overheating and potential inflammation, earth/water types, and those with earth/water imbalance, usually benefit from all three components. So the discussion on Tummo Yoga's physical exercises was saved for this chapter because earth/water types need this movement as medicine. You need motion in your ocean; you need rumble in your jungle. As you work with visualization, breath, and physical exercises, the tummo fire will stimulate and regulate your body temperature, which benefits body, energy, and mind. On a physical level, tummo fire combats earth/water's cold-natured disorders like sluggish digestion, tingly limbs, and zero libido so you can return to the land of the living and poop and move and make love. On an energetic level, tummo fire melts the stagnant knots of toxins, returning you to your primordial flow of equanimity and spaciousness. On a mental level, tummo fire invites the happy hormones that usher the dawning of bodhicitta. With tummo fire stoked, body, energy, and mind shake off the frozen, depressed, zombie state revealing your warm, connected, awakened human nature.

The physical exercises of Tummo Yoga are called Trulkhor, which means magic wheel. Have you ever seen those people spinning fire wheels? There are actually two separate fires on either end of one stick, but they spin the stick fast enough to create a continuous circle of fire. Through Trulkhor, you become that circle of fire. You reconnect all your parts to recreate a whole being. You call back your life force. You reclaim your original state. You reveal the magic wheel that you are. This is why Tibetan yogas are very dynamic. Maybe you have experience with popular yoga that feels relaxing as you do it. Trulkhor is not like that. It is not sexy and stretchy. It is fast and focused. You are clearing stagnant channels and untying toxic knots—this requires rapid, repetitive movement with breath retention. Trulkhor can feel extremely challenging, especially when you encounter these exercises in adulthood as many Westerners do. Ideally, you practice Trulkhor early in your tantric path, which means ages eight to sixteen in Tibet. But don't get discouraged and think that you are too late to do Trulkhor. You can always do it in a soft and gentle way. Also, you might surprise yourself, because it is not you that is doing Trulkhor.

Tummo Yoga is a completion stage practice, and, as such, you generate as a deity. This is one way in which Tummo Yoga differs from Nejang Yoga. You can do Nejang Yoga as yourself, which is why it was presented as a pre-empowerment practice. For Tummo Yoga, you generate as a wrathful, fiery-red female deity—and if anyone can do anything, it's her. She is beyond space and time. She eats your meat for breakfast and has no bones about it. And she lives within you. You visualize yourself as the fiery-red female deity for the entire time you practice Trulkhor. So, you see, it really is not you that is doing the practice. It is the fiery-red female deity—who lives within us all. And, of course, you can use another deity—whatever works for you. Practicing the physical exercises as a deity is very powerful training for the brain. So don't worry if you can't do the exercises well or you can't do the visualization well. Just do the practice every day, even for ten to twenty minutes. When you regularly generate as the deity and perform the exercises, your brain takes a break from being you to be deity-you. You have this inner feeling that your body is becoming flexible and the exercises are becoming easier—because your brain thinks you are the deity. And the deity doesn't have arthritis or sciatica; the deity doesn't feel old and overweight. The fiery-red female deity is flying like a magic wheel, and so are you. You are not delusional and hallucinating. You are relaxing and rewiring your brain. Your ordinary blah blahs have left the building. You are flowing and free.

This lifetime's meat is only a superficial aspect of you. It may sound disparaging to call your body meat, but, in tantra, being meat is a precious pathway to transcending meat. Right now, you are confused about the meat. You have a sense that there is physically more to you than meat, but being meat is all you know. Still, you think there is something else going on here. So you stew over the meat. You alternate between parading and hiding the meat, indulging and denying the meat, praising and blaming the meat. It is this hamster wheel of meat mania that disparages the meat. You are not treating the meat with respect; you are not letting the meat show you its potential.

In the same way that you can discover selflessness through the self, you can discover transcendence through embodiment. Within your physical body, you have an energy body. This is the body of light that you come to know whenever you generate as a buddha or deity. Then, through Tummo Yoga as the initial completion stage practice, you come to know this light body as a bliss body. It is a body of enjoyment. The enjoyment body carries you into the infinite-space body. At the conclusion of practice, you dissolve the visualization and rest with an unprecedented sense of wholeness and connection and completion. This is uncreated freedom. This is what you are. This cannot be destroyed. The problem is that you get stuck in the physical body and forget how to access infinite space. But if you practice and practice within this body, you will find it— Buddha Nature.

When earth/water types are balanced, you are skilled at holding space. If you move and heat your meat with Tummo Yoga, you can actually become space. And if you think holding space is beneficial for self and other, wait until you see what being space does for you and our world. It is okay if right now you are experiencing your body as dense, solid, and separate. Through practice, you can experience your body as light, then bliss, then space. This is the spiritual journey into transcendence, and it happens in your boring old body. For this transformation, it doesn't matter what your body looks like or what your body is wearing or what other bodies are around your body or what names you give your body or what identities your body carries or what trauma your body has undergone or what sights your body has seen or what you love about your body or what you hate about your body or who follows your body or who ignores your body or who desires your body or who disparages your body. You have a body? Good, that body works for this process. With your body, you can go beyond your body. Within this mundane piece of meat, you can become limitless loving space. In this framing, space is the feminine principle of wisdom and love is the masculine principle of compassion. So the flow of Tummo Yoga lifts you into the two wings of Buddhadharma. You fly in the space you are.

Clear Light Yoga

Clear Light Yoga is the yoga of the deep sleep state. Now you get to dive down. All this talk of flowing and fasting and lightening up—kiss it goodnight. With Clear Light Yoga, you sink into sleep. You use your slumber superpower to uncover space. You do not mess around with dreams to discover the nonduality of subject and object. Instead, you dissolve into the nondual source—the clear light.

Often, spiritual people feel guilty about sleeping, thinking they need to be up at the crack of dawn to do spiritual stuff. But sleep is vital to our physical and spiritual health. We need nighttime sleep of seven to nine hours and daytime power naps of five to fifteen minutes. Sleep improves the immune system and brain function. It stabilizes emotions and weight. It is rejuvenating and anti-aging. It prevents chronic disease. All of your problems—mental and physical—get worse with lack of sleep. So, too, all of your problems are helped by proper sleep. This means that sleep can clear physical toxins and mental toxins—including ignorance, desire, anger, pride, jealousy, and so on. This is especially true of the deep sleep state where you completely cease the confusion of self-other.

But you don't need to be convinced of sleep's beauty, do you? You have a gift, good earth/water one. You can go down hard. Your struggle is waking up. But if you can spiritually wake up during sleep, you will also physically wake up more easily. You won't be so susceptible to the torpor of earth/water imbalance. So if you are a deep sleeper and do not remember your dreams, just focus on Clear Light Yoga. If you do remember some dreams, work with Dream Yoga for three months and then move into Clear Light Yoga.

You can practice Clear Light Yoga during your nighttime sleep and daytime power naps. As always, the practice requires transmission and instruction, but we can briefly look at the process and potential of Clear Light Yoga. First, the entry is similar to Dream Yoga. Having practiced Guru Yoga during the day, you lie on your right side and place the guru in your heart as you go to sleep. You see Yuthok as dark blue and sitting on a blue lotus in your heart chakra. Dream Yoga uses the color red because the doorway to the practice is in your throat chakra. Clear Light Yoga uses the color blue because the doorway to the practice is in your heart chakra. But, as always, you can use any guru and any color you would like. With the guru in your heart, you say a prayer to accomplish Clear Light Yoga and then you repeat the mantra, audibly or silently—A NU TA RA HUNG. Blue light radiates from the guru's heart and reaches all sentient beings. The entire universe dissolves into blue light, and the light returns to the guru's heart. Then the light radiates again from the guru's heart, offering to all the buddhas. They also dissolve into blue light, and the light returns to the guru's heart. Then you go to sleep.

But where do you go when you go to sleep? What is the clear light of deep sleep? Normally, you don't notice the clear light. Falling asleep usually feels like fainting. You fall into a dark space without awareness of even falling. While in deep sleep, there is no feeling of time. When you wake up, it is like waking up from a coma. You feel like you missed something. You feel like you were gone for minutes not hours. You remember that you fell asleep, and you know you are awake now. But you have no idea what happened during deep sleep. There is a gap. The gap feels like darkness. The gap feels like a black hole. With Clear Light Yoga, you discover that the gap is actually full of light.

You have inner light. This may be why some people do drugs—so they can see inner lights. But you don't need the stimulation of substances to know your inner light. When you dream, there is light in your dream. You see sunlight, colors, and forms. When you daydream, there is light in those dreams, too. You have visions in your imagination. When you close your eyes, you might see light. When you hit your head, you might see light. If you are really lucky, when you have an orgasm, you might see light. The light, the bliss, the mantra AHHHH! All of these lights—of dreams, daydreams, injury, orgasm—are signs of inner light. You are introduced to this inner light through empowerments and Guru Yoga. As you know, the light of your heart chakra is blue. With Concise Guru Yoga, we talked about how the opening of the heart chakra allows for the opening of all the chakras; it allows for the untying of all the knots and clearing of all stagnation. This blue light of the heart chakra is your clear light. If you fall asleep consciously, slowly slowly, then you are not falling into a dark space; you are dissolving into the clear light. But this brilliant clear light of your heart chakra is only the baby clear light.

The moment when you die you will meet the mother clear light. Many people who have had near-death experiences talk about the light. They go through light tunnels. They fly through lights. They meet light beings. It's all about the light. Different spiritual paths and religions have different words for this light, and that is all good. In Tantric Buddhism, this light is your ultimate nature. Your organic true being is light and bliss. When you die, your elements dissolve—earth into water, water into fire, fire into wind, wind into space. As you take your final breath, you feel the lights coming. You may see very bright white light and then strong red light and then dark blue space. After that comes the mother clear light. When the mother clear light manifests… words cannot do it justice. Many people have a swooning experience because the light is so powerful. If you faint and fail to recognize the mother clear light, you enter the bardo—the wandering before you are habitually pulled into your next life. But if you recognize the mother clear light—in any name you want to call it—you will be spiritually liberated. The baby clear light reunites with the mother clear light. That is the final nonduality.

In Clear Light Yoga, you are training for this moment of meeting the mother clear light. You are learning how to be aware of the baby clear light at sleep so you can be aware of the mother clear light at death. Because the mother clear light is massive and shocking, you need a lifetime of practice to be present at the end of life. Don't worry though; if you miss the mother clear light, there are other moments in the bardo to spiritually liberate. But maybe you won't need to make that journey. Maybe you can learn how to recognize the baby clear light when you fall asleep so you can embrace the mother clear light upon death.

It is so special and wonderful that deep sleep is found within the 84,000 medicines. All too often spiritual paths scold humans for sleeping. But with Tantric Buddhism, sleep can become meditation. This is especially good news for earth/water types who generally love to sleep. Whenever you want to sleep—nighttime or daytime—remember to see the blue light in your heart as you fall asleep. If you can't remember the specifics of the visualization and mantra, let it all go and just focus on the blue light in your heart chakra. The key is to stay mindful as you fall asleep.

Of course, as it goes with any meditation, staying mindful is the trickiest part of Clear Light Yoga. Right before you fall asleep, you are like a little drop of water that is starting to dissolve into the ocean. But often you resist dissolving. You feel so tired, but the drop's I, I, I is still thinking about I stuff—because the drop has had a busy day with the Eight Worldly Concerns. The drop has been worrying about its image and reputation. The drop has been worrying about its bank account and career goals. The drop has been worrying about its ass and wrinkles. The drop has been worrying about its sex life and lack of sex life. The drop has been worrying about its anger and pain. The drop has an endless list of I, I, I issues. So the self-oriented, self-protective drop does not really want to dissolve into the ocean of deep sleep. But impermanence will win. The ocean is calling the drop. Once the drop falls into the ocean, the drop's sense of self dissolves. The drop's hallucination of other dissolves. Without self and other, the drop's concerns entirely dissolve. The drop finally shuts up and doesn't say I. The drop has become the ocean and it feels so good—for a time. Then the drop becomes a bubble that sees the rest of the ocean and gets scared. The bubble state is the dream state with its dramas and traumas that mirror daily life. The ocean is the clear light state without dualism or dreams—there the drop is blissfully nondual.

We have a Tibetan expression that says day and night is like a wheel. Whatever you do in one, you will do in the other. If you become well trained in Clear Light Yoga, your nighttime and your daytime will all become blissfully nondual. It all becomes the baby clear light. The baby clear light is so beautiful; it is like infinite beautiful blue space. It is calm, silent, and profound. We think we need to go outside to see the Milky Way, but your inner milky way is much more powerful than that. And that's only the baby clear light.

For Tantric Buddhist practitioners, death is something you prepare for so much that when the moment arrives you are kind of happy and excited. You have been rehearsing for so long. Now is the performance. Yes, I'm dying, yay. You relax, stop breathing, and meet your mom.

POST-EMPOWERMENT PRACTICE – GREAT PERFECTION

Ati Yoga

Ati Yoga means utmost yoga, and it is the antidote to ignorance. Ati Yoga is simple and direct. Ati Yoga is beyond words. So there isn't much to say here.

In that vein, there is an expression worth contemplating when approaching Ati Yoga: Dharma says, "Some people talk about me, but I don't know them." It is a big issue—the ones who talk about dharma but dharma doesn't know them. Often, supposed Ati Yoga and Mahamudra practitioners think they have an advanced view and are superior to others. They read about many things and talk about many things. Then they get lost in these things.

Here is how it should be: The more you meditate, the more you understand, and the more you are quiet.

If the more you meditate, then the more you talk about everything, it means something is wrong. The solution is probably that you need to do more Guru Yoga. You need spiritual blessings to practice the Buddhadharma.

Indeed, to practice Ati Yoga, you need a guru—a teacher. Ati Yoga involves an introduction to your true nature. This introduction must come from a qualified master, and, to receive this introduction, you must be dedicated to becoming enlightened for the benefit of all beings. This is the only way because devotion and altruism open the door for the introduction. The result of the introduction may be liberation from samsara and nirvana—no more cycling between hope and fear. However, for the introduction to take effect, you must meditate. Otherwise, it is like holding the medicine in your hand but never swallowing it down. And, in that case, all you have are nice words for all your talking. If you do take the medicine and meditate, you will meet with your true nature, your fresh awareness, your original state—nudi e crudi.

You can recognize true practitioners of Ati Yoga because, in addition to being quiet, they tend to be joyful, simple, and humble. Some of the best examples are the Tibetan Buddhist masters who experienced the unspeakable in recent history. They suffered physically in such severe ways—and still, these masters were so happy. They were always smiling, laughing, and telling jokes. They were saving their nearly nonexistent food to give to others. They modeled that the physical condition is only a condition; it is not our ultimate nature. Our ultimate nature is freedom. It is the inherent freedom that arises from realizing the wisdom of emptiness. And, as discussed, this wisdom begets compassion. Many elderly Tibetans said they felt so fortunate to experience the unspeakable alongside these great masters. They learned from these masters directly without even texts between them. There were even masters who chose to remain in horrific situations when they no longer had to—they knew people were suffering there, and they wanted to be with them and support them. In our hometown, there was a story about a yogi who voluntarily spent his whole life in these horrific situations because he wanted to help others. That is Ati Yoga.

The founder of Tibetan Buddhism, Guru Rinpoche, is often quoted as saying that when you realize your true nature, your view is as vast as the sky but your conduct is as fine as flour.

DEDICATION

At the end of all Tantric Buddhist practices, it is customary to say a dedication prayer. Generally speaking, this prayer dedicates your practice to be of benefit to all beings. In this lineage, you request that this practice helps you quickly achieve the same enlightened state as Yuthok, and through this may you bring all beings into this state of enlightenment.

Without the dedication prayer, your practice is like a drop of water that falls in the dirt and dries up. With the dedication prayer, your practice is like a drop of water that falls in the ocean and continues to be of benefit evermore.

On that note, thank you for reading this chapter. Regardless of whether you explore this spiritual path, may the commentary on these practices be of great benefit to you and all those you encounter. May you be well and rest easy. May you flow through life like the waves upon the shore that you are.

Conclusion

In Sowa Rigpa, we talk about the eight qualities of water. It is sweet, cool, soft, light, clear, clean, gentle in the throat, and soothing for the stomach. It is refreshing and delicious. But these days, we can't taste water. It doesn't taste like anything to us. It tastes like something is missing. We need to add bubbles, mint, lime, sugar, rum—next thing you know, you have a mojito.

But what if you were in the forest. You've been walking for a while. Your legs are tired. You're a little hot and sweaty. You're a little hungry and thirsty. Then you hear the unmistakable sound of flowing water nearby. You feel a primal pick-me-up. After a few more turns on the trail, you see it—water running down the face of a rock, cascading into a mountain stream. You reach your hand down to make a cup, collect a bit of fresh water in your palm, bring it to your lips, and it's so sweet. It is perfect just as it is. You take a seat on a rock and feel its bumpy-but-balanced support. A cool breeze tickles your skin and enlivens your entire being. The warm sun, still high in the sky, promises a few more hours of adventure. You feel grateful for this space. There is joy in your journey.

You are the forest. Your thoughts, your feelings, your speech, your movements—they are wind, fire, earth, and water enjoying the space of being. It is perfect just as it is. The issue is that we don't know we are the forest. How could we? We have been stuffed into bonsai pots of self, covered in layers of conditioning, constrained by the normalized cult of culture. We think we need to be mojitos, adding external, artificial, and superficial ingredients like drama, distraction, success, and stimulants. Even in spirituality, we are always looking for stronger and better practices. When all we need to do is remember that we are the forest—the play of perfectly pure interdependent elements.

The Buddha said wake up. Wake up to your true nature. You are loving kindness, compassion, joy, and equanimity. You are light, free, transcendent, and nondual. You are the union of bliss and emptiness.

You are the wings of wisdom and compassion. You are limitless loving space. The treasures, teachings, practices, and path presented in this book will introduce you to your true nature. This medicine will wake you up. Call the medicine whatever you want—religion, philosophy, science, spirituality. The medicine doesn't care about names. The medicine is only here for healing.

Liberation is in your hands, but you need to put down your phone to find it. You need to break out of the bonsai pot, leave the palace, and navigate the forest on your own two feet. Your life is precious and impermanent. Don't waste your incredible human intelligence running in the hamster wheel. With the power of cause and effect, you can create whatever you want. For the benefit of us all, please put an end to the suffering of self and other.

"Liberation is in your hands."

- Dr. Nida Chenagtsang

Appendix

Wind

Ngöndro – nourishes imbalanced wind

Calm Abiding Meditation – quiets and settles the mind

Three-Part Purification Breathing – releases desire

Mantra healing – protects the mind and balances wind by gathering scattered energy

Outer Guru Yoga – builds connection to the teacher and builds self-confidence

Illusory Body Yoga – releases self-image and body-image issues

Karmamudra – transforms mundane sexual desire into spiritual liberation

Fire

Ngöndro – detoxes imbalanced fire

Thinking Meditation – transforms thoughts into wisdom

Three-Part Purification Breathing – releases anger

Mantra healing – protects the mind and balances fire by expelling aggressive energy

Inner Guru Yoga – builds connection to the teacher and the teacher within

Tummo Yoga – balances fire through homeopathy of heat cures heat

Dream Yoga – leverages vivid and lucid dreaming to master the mind, life, and bardo

Mahamudra – transforms emotional waves into awakening

Earth/Water

Ngöndro – creates flow for imbalanced earth/water

Eliminating Obstacles – eliminates obstacles in ordinary life
and spiritual practice

Nejang Yoga – heals mind, body, and energy through accessible yoga

Three-Part Purification Breathing – releases ignorance

Mantra healing – protects the mind and balances earth/water
by moving stuck energy

Concise Guru Yoga – combines all the Guru Yogas and opens
the heart chakra

Tummo Yoga – balances earth/water by warming and moving stagnant
energy

Clear Light Yoga – leverages deep sleep for meditation and prepares
one for death

Ati Yoga – dispels ignorance to reveal the nature of mind

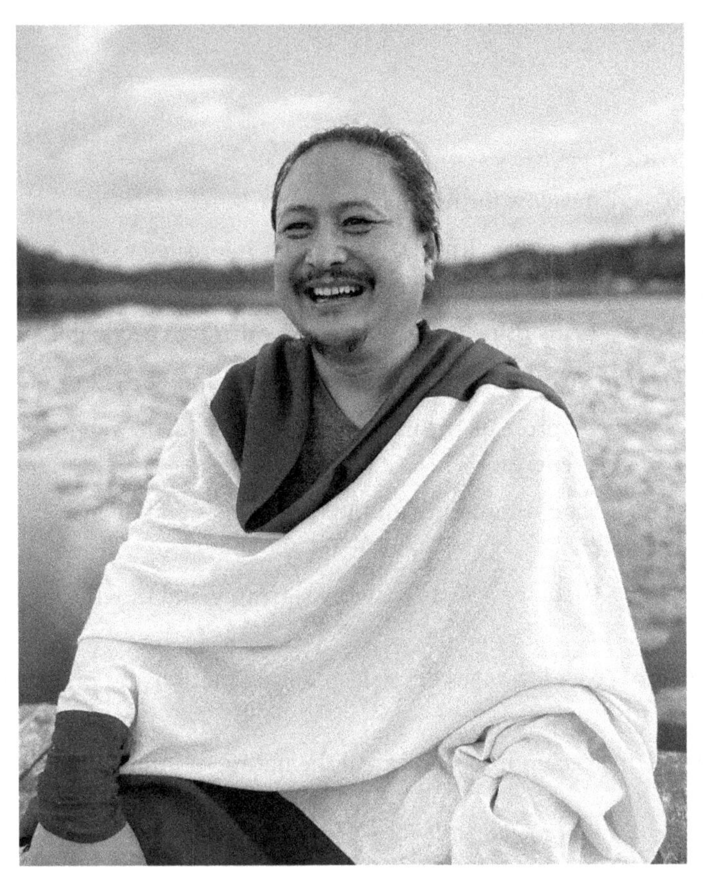

About the Author

Born in Amdo, Malho, in Northeastern Tibet, Dr. Nida began his early studies of Sowa Rigpa at the local Tibetan medical hospital. Later, he was awarded a scholarship to enter the Lhasa Mentsikhang or Tibetan Medical University, where he completed his degree in 1996, with practical training at the Tibetan Medicine hospitals in Lhasa and Lhoka. Alongside his medical education, Dr. Nida trained in Vajrayana with teachers from every school of Tibetan Buddhism. In particular, he trained in the Longchen Nyingthig tradition of the Nyingma school with his root guru Ani Ngawang Gyaltsen and in the Dudjom Tersar tradition with Chönyi Rinpoche and Semo Dechen Yudrön. He received complete instruction in the Yuthok Nyingthig lineage, the unique spiritual tradition of Tibetan Medicine, from his teachers Khenpo Tsultrim Gyaltsen and Khenchen Troru Tsenam, and was requested to continue the Yuthok Nyingthig lineage by Jamyang Rinpoche of the Rebkong ngakpa and ngakma (i.e. non-monastic yogi and yogini) community.

A well-known poet in his youth, Dr. Nida later published many articles and books on Sowa Rigpa and the Yuthok Nyingthig tradition in Tibetan and English, which have been translated into several languages. He has extensively researched ancient Tibetan healing methods, and has gained acclaim in East and West for his revival of little-known Tibetan external therapies.

Dr. Nida is the Founder and Medical Director of the Sowa Rigpa Institute of Tibetan Medicine and of Sorig Khang International: Foundation for Traditional Tibetan Medicine. He is also the co-founder and principal teacher of Pure Land Farms center for Tibetan medicine, meditation, and rejuvenation in Los Angeles; and the co-founder of the International Ngakmang Institute, which was established to preserve and support the unique Rebkong non-monastic yogi and yogini culture in modern Tibetan society. In addition to his work as a physician, Dr. Nida trains students in Sowa Rigpa and the Yuthok Nyingthig tradition in over forty countries around the world.

To learn about Dr Nida's publications please visit:
www.skypressbooks.com